AF745557

IRON DEFICIENCY ANEMIA

Edited by **Luis Rodrigo**

Iron Deficiency Anemia
http://dx.doi.org/10.5772/intechopen.73922
Edited by Luis Rodrigo

Contributors

Roberto Miniero, Valentina Talarico, Maria Concetta Galati, Laura Giancotti, Paola Saracco, Giuseppe Raiola, Yangho Kim, Francesco Fedele, Massimo Mancone, Carmen Caira, Alessandra Cinque, Viviana Maestrini, Mario Alberto Ruiz-Lopez, Ramon Rodriguez-Macias, Elia Hermila Valdes-Miramontes, Елена Zhukovskaya, Alexander Karelin, Alexander Rumyantsev, Claudia Burz, Andrei Cismaru, Vlad Vasile Pop, Anca Bojan

© The Editor(s) and the Author(s) 2019
The rights of the editor(s) and the author(s) have been asserted in accordance with the Copyright, Designs and Patents Act 1988. All rights to the book as a whole are reserved by INTECHOPEN LIMITED. The book as a whole (compilation) cannot be reproduced, distributed or used for commercial or non-commercial purposes without INTECHOPEN LIMITED's written permission. Enquiries concerning the use of the book should be directed to INTECHOPEN LIMITED rights and permissions department (permissions@intechopen.com).
Violations are liable to prosecution under the governing Copyright Law.

(cc) BY

Individual chapters of this publication are distributed under the terms of the Creative Commons Attribution 3.0 Unported License which permits commercial use, distribution and reproduction of the individual chapters, provided the original author(s) and source publication are appropriately acknowledged. If so indicated, certain images may not be included under the Creative Commons license. In such cases users will need to obtain permission from the license holder to reproduce the material. More details and guidelines concerning content reuse and adaptation can be found at http://www.intechopen.com/copyright-policy.html.

Notice

Statements and opinions expressed in the chapters are these of the individual contributors and not necessarily those of the editors or publisher. No responsibility is accepted for the accuracy of information contained in the published chapters. The publisher assumes no responsibility for any damage or injury to persons or property arising out of the use of any materials, instructions, methods or ideas contained in the book.

First published in London, United Kingdom, 2019 by IntechOpen
IntechOpen is the global imprint of INTECHOPEN LIMITED, registered in England and Wales, registration number: 11086078, The Shard, 25th floor, 32 London Bridge Street
London, SE19SG – United Kingdom
Printed in Croatia

British Library Cataloguing-in-Publication Data
A catalogue record for this book is available from the British Library

Additional hard copies can be obtained from orders@intechopen.com

Iron Deficiency Anemia, Edited by Luis Rodrigo
p. cm.
Print ISBN 978-1-78985-443-5
Online ISBN 978-1-78985-444-2
eBook (PDF) ISBN 978-1-83880-642-2

We are IntechOpen, the world's leading publisher of Open Access books

Built by scientists, for scientists

4,100+
Open access books available

116,000+
International authors and editors

120M+
Downloads

151
Countries delivered to

Our authors are among the
Top 1%
most cited scientists

12.2%
Contributors from top 500 universities

WEB OF SCIENCE™

Selection of our books indexed in the Book Citation Index
in Web of Science™ Core Collection (BKCI)

Interested in publishing with us?
Contact book.department@intechopen.com

Numbers displayed above are based on latest data collected.
For more information visit www.intechopen.com

For EU product safety concerns:
IN TECH d.o.o., Prolaz Marije Krucifikse Kozulić 3, 51000 Rijeka, Croatia,
info@intechopen.com or visit our website at intechopen.com.

Meet the editor

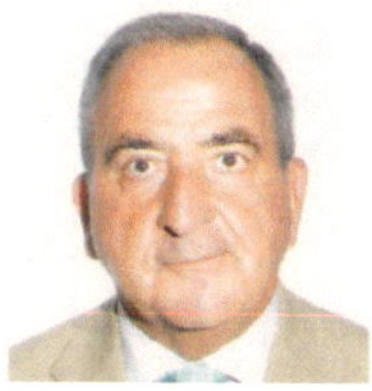

Dr. Luis Rodrigo MD is actually Emeritus Professor of Medicine at the University of Oviedo (Spain). He has been the Chief of Gastroenterology Service at the HUCA Hospital in Oviedo, for more than 40 years. He obtained the PhD at 1975 and has developed a long Teaching and Research Career. He has published a total of 575 scientific papers, 297 written in English and the rest in Spanish. He has participated as main investigator in a total of 45 Clinical Trials and has directed 40 Doctoral Thesis. He has contributed actively to the formation of around one hundred specialist in Gastroenterology working in his Hospital and another hospitals in Spain and aboad. He has written around of 35 chapters in books of several subjects and has been the editor of 22 books in his speciality and related diseases.

Contents

Preface

It is estimated that one-third of the world's population is anemic, the majority being due to iron deficiency (ID). This great health problem affects approximately to more than 2 billion people worldwide, and IDA remains the main cause of anemia, as confirmed by the analysis of a large number of reports on the burden of disease in near two hundred countries, performed in the last twenty years and by a survey on the burden of anemia in persons at risk, such as preschool children and young women.

This situation is applied to the reduction of iron stores that precedes to overt iron deficiency anemia (IDA) or persists without progression. This is a more severe condition, in which low levels of iron are associated with anemia and the presence of microcytic hypochromic red cells. The estimated prevalence of ID worldwide, is twice as high the IDA. The diagnosis and treatment of this condition needs clearly to be improved.

Iron is a metal compound crucial to biologic functions, including respiration, energy production, DNA synthesis, and cell proliferation. The human body has evolved to conserve iron in several ways, including the recycling of iron after the breakdown of red cells and the retention of iron in the absence of an excretion mechanism. However, since excess levels of iron can be toxic, its absorption is limited to 1 to 2 mg daily, and most of the iron needed daily (about 25 mg per day) is provided through recycling by macrophages that phagocytate senescent erythrocytes. The latter two mechanisms are controlled by the hormone hepcidin, which maintains total-body iron within normal ranges, avoiding both iron deficiency and excess.

Prevention programs have decreased rates of IDA globally. The prevalence is now highest in Central and West Africa and South Asia. The reported prevalence of ID in the absence of dietary fortification is approximately 40% in preschool children, 30% in menstruating girls and women, and 38% in pregnant women. These rates reflect the increased physiological need for dietary iron during specific life stages according to sex.

While anemia is clearly defined according to the World Health Organization as a hemoglobin (Hb) level less than 12 g/dL in women (< 11 g/dL in pregnant women) and lower than 13 g/dL in men, the situation is ambiguous for for iron deficiency. No single test is diagnostic of ID, unless the serum ferritin is low or the percent transferrin saturation is low with an elevated total iron binding capacity

Iron deficiency anemia (IDA) is a common complication in routine clinical practice that frequently originates in the gastrointestinal (GI) tract. Patients with IDA are therefore often referred to gastroenterologists for further examination and/or treatment. This finding associated with GI disorders can substantially reduces quality of life, contribute to fatigue, and may even lead to hospitalization.

In contrast to the well-documented inflammatory bowel disease (IBD)-associated IDA prevalence data for associated with other pathological conditions of the GI tract, are sparse.

Guidelines for the diagnosis and management of anemia and iron deficiency are available for IBD, but not for other GI conditions. Overall, there are three main pathological contributors to IDA, namely chronic bleeding, malabsorption and inflammation. However, other factors, such as poor or selective diet, as well as iron malabsorption (e.g., due to decreased gastric pH) should not be neglected in patients referred for IDA assessment. This applies particularly to elderly patients.

Celiac disease (CD) is one of the most common chronic inflammatory conditions of the GI system, affecting about 1% of the population. There is a well established relationship between CD and IDA. Anemia is the most common presenting symptom of CD, found in 32%-69% of adult patients. Approximately 80% of anemic patients with CD, are also ID. In 49% of anemic patients with CD, ID was found to be the only detectable abnormality. Conversely, among patients presenting with unexplained IDA, 5% have histologically-confirmed CD. Impaired iron absorption (due to villous atrophy of the intestinal mucosa) and blood loss are important pathological contributors to anemia in CD.

Occult GI bleeding has been detected in about half of patients with CD adhering to a gluten-free diet (GFD). In some patients, nutritional deficiencies may also be a (contributing) causative factor. Inflammation is a major contributor to IDA, with interleukin (IL)-1, IL-6, IL-10, interferon (IFN)-γ and tumor necrosis factor (TNF)-α as inducers of hepcidin, the main regulator of iron homeostasis .

Accordingly, CD-related IDA, is refractory to oral iron treatment, and even after switching to a GFD, it takes 6-12 mo until most patients recover from anemia. Notably, half of patients remain iron-deficient even after 1-2 years on a GFD. The slow or lacking recovery from ID, may be due to the low absorption rate of nutritional iron (1-2 mg/d), which hinders the repletion of severely depleted iron stores, and the potentially low content of iron and other micronutrients in a GFD. Therefore, patients with CD clearly benefit from immediate intravenous iron treatment, instead of switching to intravenous iron only after (foreseeable) non-response and/or intolerance to oral iron.

Oral iron is considered the front line therapy, except for conditions such as gastric bypass, heavy uterine bleeding, inflammatory bowel disease, and hereditary hemorrhagic telangiectasia. Oral iron has many unpleasant side effects, resulting in low patient adherence. For patients intolerant of or unresponsive to, oral iron, intravenous (IV) administration is the preferred route.

While early formulations were associated with a high incidence of serious adverse events (SAEs), newer formulations are much safer with SAEs occurring very infrequently. Full replacement doses can be administered in a matter of minutes to a few hours. Nevertheless, there remains a reluctance to use IV iron due to a misunderstanding of the safety of the available formulations. Intrevenous iron is safe and effective in all clinical circumstances including pregnancy. The preponderance of published evidence suggests IV iron therapy is underutilized and IV iron should be moved forward in the treatment of ID and IDA.

Prof. Luis Rodrigo MD
Emeritus Full Professor of Medicine
University of Oviedo
Oviedo, Spain

Chapter 1

Iron-Deficiency Anemia

Claudia Burz, Andrei Cismaru, Vlad Pop and
Anca Bojan

Additional information is available at the end of the chapter

http://dx.doi.org/10.5772/intechopen.80940

Abstract

Iron is an important element in living systems as it participates in a series of metabolic processes including DNA synthesis and oxygen and electron transport. Iron deficiency is the most common cause of anemia globally being an important healthcare problem. If left untreated, iron-deficiency anemia (IDA) can cause significant morbidity and often is the result of a more serious underlying condition. Correcting iron deficiency and replenishing iron reserves are important objectives of a well-conducted treatment, but diagnosis should prompt further investigation to establish the cause for potential reversal. Age, tolerance, preferred route of administration, and severity of anemia are some of the patient's characteristics which require an individualized approach.

Keywords: anemia, iron deficiency, hemoglobin, ferritin, transferrin, hepcidin, erythropoiesis

1. Introduction

Anemia is the most common hematologic disorder, iron deficiency being the leading cause worldwide [1]. Often, anemia is the presenting sign of a more serious underlying condition which left untreated can generate consequent morbidity [2]. Likewise, it can worsen preexisting comorbidities such as cardiac and pulmonary disease. The World Health Organization (WHO) defines anemia as hemoglobin levels lower than 13 g/dL in men and 12 g/dL in women (**Table 1**) with variations in age and pregnancy. Moreover, altitude and smoking status can influence baseline hemoglobin [3, 4]. Red blood cells (RBC) are responsible for hemoglobin levels. Deficits in their production, increased destruction, or loss through bleeding are the main three mechanisms by which anemia occurs. Risk factors include female gender, extremes of

IntechOpen

© 2018 The Author(s). Licensee IntechOpen. This chapter is distributed under the terms of the Creative Commons Attribution License (http://creativecommons.org/licenses/by/3.0), which permits unrestricted use, distribution, and reproduction in any medium, provided the original work is properly cited.

Population	Mild anemia	Moderate anemia	Severe anemia
Children 0.5–4 years	10–10.9	7–9.9	<7
Children 5–11 years	11–11.4	8–10.9	<8
Children 12–14 years	11–11.9	8–10.9	<8
Pregnant women	10–10.9	7–7.9	<7
Nonpregnant women	11–11.9	8–10.9	<8
Men >15 years	11–12.9	8–10.9	<8

Levels of Hb higher than the superior value of mild anemia in each population group are considered nonanemia.

Table 1. Severity of anemia in different age groups, sex, and pregnancy status (g/dL).

age, pregnancy, and lactation. There are several types of anemia such as thalassemia, sickle cell disease, aplastic anemia, hemolytic anemia, pernicious anemia, and iron-deficiency anemia. In this chapter we will focus on a comprehensive characterization of iron-deficiency anemia (IDA).

2. Definition

Iron deficiency and IDA are serious health problems in the whole world. Iron has a vital role for many biologic functions including energy production, respiration, and cell proliferation. IDA is the end-stage result of the lack of iron in the body resulting from inadequate iron intake, increased iron loss, or excessive iron requirements [5]. As a consequence, erythropoiesis is insufficient to fulfill the body's physiologic needs. IDA diminishes working performance by constraining muscles to depend on anaerobic metabolism in order to greater attain muscle extent in contrast to healthy individuals. As a result, in affected patients the capability to perform physical labor is decreased. Furthermore, in children, both growth and learning capacities are affected.

Using the severity criteria, anemia is classified into mild (11 g/dL to normal), moderate (8 g/dL to 11 g/L), and severe (less than 8 g/dL) in adult males and adult nonpregnant females (**Table 1**) [6]. Severe anemia may produce hypoxemia enhancing the occurrence of coronary insufficiency and myocardial ischemia. Also, it may aggravate underlying cardiac and pulmonary disorders.

3. Epidemiology

Anemia is a public health problem that affects populations in both developed and undeveloped countries. According to the WHO data on the prevalence of anemia for the period between the years 1993 and 2005, anemia affects 24.8% of the population globally, which corresponds to approximately one in four people. The highest prevalence was reported in preschool-aged children (47.4%), whereas the lowest prevalence is in men (12.7%). Although the prevalence in nonpregnant women was reported at 30.2%, they represent the population group with the largest number of individuals affected (468.4 million).

WHO region	Pregnant women	Nonpregnant women	Preschool-aged children
Africa	57.1	47.5	67.6
The Americas	24.1	17.8	29.3
Southeast Asia	48.2	45.7	65.5
Europe	25.1	19.0	21.7
Eastern Mediterranean	44.2	32.4	46.7
Western Pacific	30.7	21.5	23.1
Global	**41.8**	**30.2**	**47.4**

Table 2. Prevalence of anemia in different WHO regions (in percentage (%)).

Typically, IDA represents approximately a half of all types of anemia, but the cases may vary among population groups and in different areas according to local conditions [7].

The WHO areas of Africa and Southeast Asia have the highest risk, where about two-third of preschool-aged children and half of all women are affected [8]. Prevalence in pregnant and nonpregnant women is similar in Europe and the Americas, whereas preschool children's prevalence of anemia is different in these two WHO regions (**Table 2**).

4. Etiology

The diagnosis of IDA is not sufficient; the cause of iron deficiency has to be identified. Iron deficiency occurs by disturbing the balance of iron metabolism, respectively, by **reducing the intake** or by excess **blood loss** [9].

The main situations responsible for reduced iron intake, directly or indirectly, are insufficient food intake, poor absorption, or increased requirements [10].

Regarding the insufficient food intake, this situation is rarely encountered as iron requirements are relatively low. It is more common in severe diets and vegetarianism, as heme iron, the one contained in red meat, has two times greater bioavailability than the non-heme iron from eggs and vegetables [11].

Several conditions may interfere with iron absorption, the most frequent being:

- *Achlorhydria*: prevents the absorption of nonheme iron [12].
- *Gastrectomy*: absence of gastric acidity and reduction of food contact time with digestive lining [11].
- *Long-lasting antacid treatments* reduce iron absorption [11].
- *Eating habits*: excessive consumption of tea and coffee [13].
- *Gastritis with Helicobacter pylori* [14].
- *Inflammatory diseases of the small intestine*: Crohn's disease, Whipple's disease, and celiac disease [11].

Some physiological conditions are associated with increased needs of iron and secondary apparition of IDA. Pregnancy, prematurity, twins, intense growth, and development periods during adolescence could be responsible of IDA [15–17].

The most common cause of iron deficiency remains blood loss, especially from the digestive track in men and from menstrual bleeding in women [18]:

- *Digestive conditions* may be caused by hiatal hernia, atrophic gastritis, gastric and duodenal ulcers, digestive cancers, colonic polyps, ulcerative colitis, and hemorrhoids [19–22].
- *Respiratory conditions* as lung cancers [23] or chronic infection and tuberculosis [23–24].
- *Genitourinary conditions as* menometrorrhagia, benign uterine tumors or malignant conditions, and hematuria [25–28].

Other conditions, more rarely observed, are frequent phlebotomies in blood donors, chronic kidney disease, and dialysis [29, 30].

5. Physiopathology

5.1. General aspects

IDA occurs through the disruption of iron metabolism. For a better understanding of the mechanisms by which iron balance can be altered, some important elements of iron metabolism must be taken into consideration:

1. The iron intake compensates only the physiological losses that occur through gastrointestinal epithelium exfoliation and urinary excretion [31].
2. In case of high demand or iron overload, the only regulation mechanism is represented by the digestive absorption which can be intensified or reduced. The regulation mechanism is not realized by increasing the physiological losses [32].
3. The total body iron accounts for 3–4 g in adults, and it is distributed in three compartments [33]:
    a. The functional compartment from which 70% of the total iron (2.8 g) consists in iron from hemoglobin and myoglobin and < 1% in cellular enzymes involved in oxidative metabolism: catalases, cytochromes, and myeloperoxidases.
    b. Transport compartment which represents 0.1% of the total iron, 4 mg, consists of transferrin or siderophilin. It is synthesized by the liver and has the role of transporting iron to cells. Each molecule fixes one or two atoms of trivalent iron. The evaluation of this compartment is made by:
        - Measurement of serum transferrin using immunological method.
        - Measurement of total iron-binding capacity.
        - Measurement of transferrin saturation
    c. The storage compartment represents 29% of total iron (1 g) and is contained in macrophages and hepatocytes under the form of:

- Ferritin, a water-soluble protein formed from apoferritin and iron, is found in the intracellular compartment, especially in macrophages. As the circulating iron increases, the ferritin levels also increase. A small amount is found in the blood, can be dosed, and correlates with body iron deposits.
- Hemosiderin represents a partially denatured form of ferritin. Hemosiderin found in macrophages (most of them are available by sternal bone marrow aspiration) can be identified after staining with potassium ferrocyanide (Perls staining) [34, 35].

5.2. The iron cycle

A balanced diet accounts for 10–20 mg of iron per day, of which 5% is absorbed, sufficient for covering the losses [31]. To provide the stores with the sufficient amount of iron, approximately 1 g is necessary, equivalent to the absorbed quantity in 2–3 years.

The iron intake consists of two forms [11]:

- Heme iron in red meat, more easily absorbed, in which iron exists as Fe^{2+}.
- Non-heme iron from eggs and vegetal products which is in the form of Fe^{3+}.

Iron absorption is impaired by antacids, phytates, and tannic acid. It takes place mostly in the duodenum and proximal intestine. Under conditions of rapid intestinal transit, the contact time of intestinal content with iron is reduced, and absorption is diminished. Trivalent iron is reduced to ferrous iron by the other food components or by reductase enzymes in intestinal brush cells [11, 36].

Ferrous iron is transported from the apical pole of the cell to the basal pole by the transport protein, divalent metal transporter 1 (DMT1). From this point, it is transported into the blood by ferroportin, as ferrous iron. Ferroportin's activity is regulated by hepcidin, an acute-phase protein synthesized by the liver. Hepcidin inhibits intestinal absorption of iron by accelerating degradation of ferroportin. The iron is then taken up by the transferrin. The iron-transferrin complex circulates in the blood until it interacts with specific receptors for transferrin. The complex coupled with transferrin receptors is internalized, and the iron is released and used for the synthesis of heme, while the transferrin-receptor complex reaches the cell surface where transferrin is released in the blood. At this point, a small amount of transferrin receptors can be released in the blood and can be dosed as free circulating receptors [9, 11].

In erythroid precursors, excess iron binds to apoferritin to form ferritin. This process also takes place in other cells that express transferrin receptors, for example, hepatocytes. Hepcidin inhibits iron release from macrophages. Iron incorporated in hemoglobin enters the circulation providing oxygen to tissues [37, 38].

The lifespan of a RBC is 120 days [33]. Then, erythrocytes are recognized as senescent cells by the reticuloendothelial system (RES) and hepatocytes, and as a result, they are destroyed by the phagocytes [39]. Hemoglobin is decomposed to globin and restores the deposit of amino acids. The iron is transported to the cell surface where it is taken by transferrin (iron recycling) [40].

The absorption is controlled by an active mechanism. It is influenced by several factors. RBC hyperplasia stimulates the absorption of iron, even if iron storages are normal or increased and hepcidin levels are reduced. The molecular mechanism behind is unknown. Patients with associated anemia and ineffective erythropoiesis (thalassemia intermedia) have an excessive absorption of iron. In IDA, the hepcidin level is low, and iron is more efficiently absorbed from food. During inflammation, hepcidin levels increase, due to the fact that it is an acute-phase protein. This determines macrophages to retain the iron and to reduce iron absorption, determining iron deficiency [33, 41, 42].

Ferroportin acts also on the erythrocyte precursors, promoting the export of the iron to RBC precursors (**Figure 1**) [43].

5.3. Stages of iron deficiency

The first stage of iron deficiency is the reduction of iron stores. In order to compensate the deficiency, the iron is released from the stores, initially from ferritin, which is easily available, and then from hemosiderin. Thus, iron intestinal absorption and transferrin synthesis intensify, but on the other hand, the iron saturation of transferrin is reduced, and total binding capacity of transferrin increases. At this stage, due to the mobilization of iron from the stores, the levels of circulating iron are normal [44].

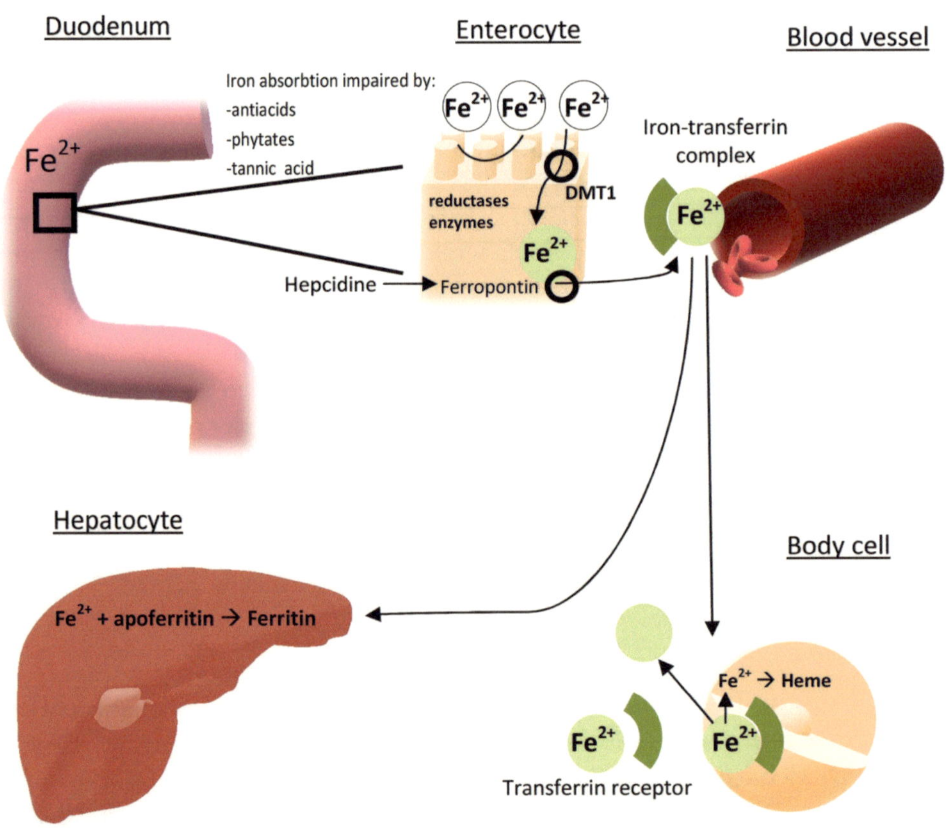

Figure 1. Schematic representation of iron circuit in the human body.

The second stage is represented by the total depletion of iron stores. At this moment the serum iron is low, but erythropoiesis is not affected [44].

The last stage is represented by the hypochromic microcytic anemia. At this stage, the quantity of iron delivered to the erythroblasts is insufficient, the synthesis of hemoglobin is reduced, and hypochromia occurs. Afterward, by enhancing the mitotic erythroblast activity, microcytosis occurs. The number of RBC is diminished, but not lower than the amount of hemoglobin. Due to the hypoxia, erythropoietin synthesis is stimulated, but the erythropoiesis cannot increase because of the low amounts of hemoglobin. Therefore, reticulocyte count will be normal or decreased. Iron deficiency causes the reduction of other body components that contain iron, such as myoglobin, cytochromes, and catalases, which are responsible for the late extrahematologic signs of iron deficiency [44, 45].

6. Clinical presentation

The clinical features of IDA depend on many factors including age group, comorbidity, anemia level, and speed of onset. Several symptoms may be present, some associated with all types of anemia such as pallor or asthenia. Other symptoms are caused by the iron deficiency that affects the epithelial cells, or in some cases, the symptoms may be caused by the disease which determined the disruption of iron metabolism.

Symptoms and signs resulting from anemia depend on the underlying cardiovascular status of the patient, most important being summarized in **Table 3**.

Depending on the underlying condition that caused the iron deficiency, the patients may present different symptoms and signs such as abdominal pain, urinary and genital symptoms, and respiratory disorders. The most frequent conditions associated with iron deficiency are gastric and duodenal ulcers; hiatal hernia; digestive carcinomas; and surgical interventions such as gastrectomy, intestinal resections, or urogenital pathology, for example, uterine fibroid, genital cancer in women, and kidney diseases that cause hematuria [46–48].

Symptoms caused by tissue hypoxia	Symptoms caused by the heart or lung adaption to hypoxia	Symptoms and signs due to iron deficiency
• Pallor	• Tachycardia	• Dysphagia
• Fatigue	• Tachypnea	• Plummer-Vinson syndrome
• General weakness	• Dyspnea	• Nail changes, koilonychia
• Headache		• Friable hair
• Vertigo		• Angular cheilitis
• Tinnitus		• Stomatitis
• Angina pectoris		
• Intermittent claudication		
• Poor appetite		

Table 3. Symptoms associated with iron deficiency.

7. Diagnosis of IDA

Diagnosis of IDA involves reduced hemoglobin levels and disturbed iron parameters. The initial evaluation includes a complete blood count (CBC), reticulocyte count, peripheral blood smear, and serum iron parameters. The CBC is useful in determining the concentration of hemoglobin, the mean corpuscular volume, and the average size of RBC.

The CBC highlights:

- Low hemoglobin level.
- The number of RBC decreases later but proportionally less than the hemoglobin levels.
- The mean corpuscular volume (MCV) is <80 fl and HEM <27 pg.%. So, anemia is a hypochromic microcytic because of the decreased hemoglobin level.
- Reticulocyte count is normal or slightly elevated.
- On the blood smear, erythrocytes have a fading center with a periphery of hemoglobin (anulocytes).

RBC dimensions are variable, unequal in size and generally smaller, this situation being known as anisocytosis. This reflects an increased red blood cell distribution width index (RDW). The number of white blood cells and their morphology is normal, whereas moderate thrombocytosis is frequently encountered, but it resolves after the correction of iron deficiency.

After the diagnosis of anemia, one should proceed to explore the iron metabolism. Evaluation of serum ferritin is the most used diagnostic test, but its level increases in inflammatory disease and in old persons. For the diagnosis of IDA, some parameters as transferrin, soluble transferrin receptor (sTfR), and the soluble transferrin receptor/ferritin index could be useful. The accuracy of some of these markers is limited being influenced by many other conditions, especially the level of serum ferritin. The most used parameter, serum ferritin level, can be increased in acute or chronic inflammation, old persons, chronic infection, or malignancy status. One more sensitive parameter for IDA diagnosis is soluble transferrin receptor (sTfR) that remains unaffected by inflammatory states being an indirect measure of erythropoiesis.

Usually, in clinical practice, the diagnosis of IDA includes low hemoglobin level, low transferrin saturation (<15%), low levels of serum ferritin (<30 ug/dl), and high total iron binding capacity (>13.1 umol/l). Another method of exploring iron reserves consists in the appreciation of the medullary reticulocytes through a medullary smear (bone marrow cytology) and Perls staining. This highlights the absence of hemosiderin (iron reserves), the absence of sideroblasts (lack of iron in erythroblasts), and the absence of siderocytes (lack of iron in red blood cells). This exam is not routinely required.

Finally, after establishing the diagnosis of IDA, an iron deficiency cause should be investigated, as the most common cause in men is digestive losses and in women genital losses. These investigations should include gynecological examination and the exploration of the digestive tract: gastroscopy, colonoscopy, and other investigations according to specific elements identified in the medical history and physical exam [33, 49–51].

http://dx.doi.org/10.5772/intechopen.80940

8. Differential diagnosis

The differential diagnosis of IDA should be made with other forms of microcytic anemia (see **Table 4**):

(a) Anemia from chronic disease where one of the main mechanisms is the blockage of iron in its reserves, as in macrophages and the inability to be used in erythropoiesis.

Common elements:

- Hypochromic microcytic anemia.
- Serum iron is low.

Elements of differential diagnosis:

- The total capacity of iron attachment is normal or decreased (overall amounts of iron are not decreased).
- Ferritin is normal or increased (acute-phase protein, iron reserves are increased).
- Signs of the underlying disease are present: chronic infections, collagen diseases, neoplasia, etc.
- Biological markers of inflammation are present: fibrinogen, C-reactive protein, alpha-2-globulin, etc.)

(b) Thalassemia minor

Common elements:

- Hypochromic microcytic anemia.

Elements of differential diagnosis:

- The number of RBC is twofold higher.
- The RDW (erythrocyte distribution index) is normal.

Anemia from chronic disease
Chronic inflammatory disorders
Chronic infections
Autoimmune diseases
Kidney diseases
Cancer
Thalassemia minor
Sideroblastic anemia

Table 4. Differential diagnosis of iron-deficiency anemia.

Smear shows frequent red blood cells with basophile points and bull's-eye erythrocytes (codocytes):

- Serum iron is normal.
- Ferritin is normal or increased.

The diagnosis of certainty is determined by hemoglobin electrophoresis: increased amount of fetal hemoglobin (HbF) or hemoglobin A2.

(c) Sideroblastic anemia

Common elements:

- Hypochromic microcytic anemia.

Elements of differential diagnosis:

- Normal or increased serum iron.
- Increased level of ferritin.
- There is no chronic disease or biological signs of inflammation.
- Bone marrow cytology with Perls staining: ring-shaped sideroblasts (the iron is placed in the mitochondria with a ring around its core).

Difficulties in diagnosis:

- Previous treatment with iron supplements.
- Association with other deficits.
- Association with an anemia from chronic diseases [52–54].

9. Treatment

9.1. General aspects

Iron-deficiency anemia and/or iron deficiency should be treated, regardless of the presence or absence of symptoms. The correction of anemia is vital; depending on its severity, anemia could trigger cardiovascular complications, sometimes severe [55, 56].

Treatment of IDA has two major objectives:

1. Substitution treatment with iron products, aiming to correct anemia and replenishing the iron reserves
2. The detection and treatment of the underlying cause of anemia

9.2. Iron therapy

The treatment of iron deficiency is either enteral or parenteral.

Intramuscular administration of iron is rarely used due to local complications such as pain at administration site, uneven absorption, skin pigmentation, and even development of sarcomas at the injection site as some authors have reported [57, 58].

Transdermal administration has been experimented in animal models, but there is no evidence that it would be effective and safe in humans [59].

9.2.1. *Oral iron therapy*

9.2.1.1. *Treatment with oral iron products*

Treatment with oral iron products is preferable due to the low cost and lack of anaphylactic side effect. Usually, it is used to treat iron-deficiency anemia in children and adolescents.

Indication:

The main indications of oral iron are treatment of IDA, treatment of iron deficiency, and prophylaxis of iron deficiency in subjects with high needs such as pregnant women, adolescents, and preterm children.

A wide range of iron products is available in forms of tablets or liquid. Liquid iron products have the advantage of allowing titration of the dose. The most commonly used oral iron products are polysaccharide iron complex, ferrous gluconate, ferrous sulfate, and ferrous fumarate.

Dosage:

Regarding the dosage, various over-the-counter tablets exist depending on the products, but generally, there are no differences between these products in effectiveness or adverse events. The daily dose needed to correct iron deficiency depends on age, iron deficiency, and urgency. In general, daily dose for the correction of IDA with oral products is 150–200 mg elemental iron. Reports show that this dose taken every other day is most effective and has a better absorption and fewer side effects [60, 61].

Toxicity of iron products is more important in elderly patients, so doses are smaller. In a randomized study of 90 patients, of over 80 years old with iron deficiency, doses of 10, 15, or 150 mg for 2 months were equally effective [62].

The bioavailability and absorption of oral iron products may be influenced by food (e.g., phytates, phosphates, and tannins can bind iron and prevent absorption) or by drugs which diminish gastric secretion (antacids, histamine receptor inhibitors, proton pump inhibitors, etc.) reducing the absorption of iron. This is why iron products are administered 2 hours before and 4 hours after the administration of antacid absorption of iron as ferrous iron depending on acidic environment.

In general, iron product administration is associated with acidic foods (orange juice) or vitamin C to promote iron absorption, but there are no studies that show a positive effect of vitamin C in the absorption of iron [63].

There is no consensus on the duration of treatment with oral iron products. Some experts end treatment after correcting anemia to allow early detection of secondary anemia, due to recurrent blood loss. Others recommend continuing treatment for 6 months after correction of anemia in order to supplement iron reserves. Generally, 6 weeks of treatment are needed to correct anemia, followed by 6 months to replenish the reserves.

Side effect of oral therapy:

Concerning the side effects of oral iron therapy, the most common side effects involving gastrointestinal tract are metallic taste, nausea, flatulence, constipation, diarrhea, epigastric pain, and/or vomit. Black stools create anxiety as they may be misinterpreted as gastrointestinal bleeding.

Some measures can be taken in order to diminish iron side effects and increase tolerability as increasing the time between administrations (given every other day, not daily), changing diet (concomitant administration of food, even if absorption is reduced), reducing daily dose of elemental iron, switching from tablets to liquid preparations that allow titration of doses, or switching from tables to IV administration.

9.2.1.2. Treatment with IV iron products

Indication:

There are some specific indications for IV administered iron products when oral administration is inefficient or contraindicated (see **Table 5**):

- Patients who do not tolerate oral products due to gastrointestinal symptoms especially elderly, pregnant women, and patients with gastrointestinal disorders for which the administration of these products may aggravate symptoms.
- Patients with uncontrollable chronic blood loss that cannot be corrected by oral treatment (Rendu-Osler disease and other vascular malformations, cancer, etc.).
- Patients who have undergone surgery of the digestive tract that affects the absorption: gastrectomies and surgical bypass.
- Patients with pathology associating malabsorption or inflammatory disease like celiac disease, Whipple disease, etc.
- Patients who require replenishing iron reserves in one to two sessions instead of prolonged treatments.

Oral therapy	Parenteral administration
Indication	**Indication**
• Treatment of iron deficiency and prophylaxis of iron deficiency in subjects with high needs such as pregnant women, adolescents, and children	• Intolerance or conditions associated with malabsorption of oral products • Uncontrollable chronic blood loss • Patients who require replenishing iron reserves in one to two sessions instead of prolonged treatments
Side effects	**Side effects**
Gastrointestinal disorders: • Nausea • Flatulence • Constipation • Diarrhea • Epigastric pain • Vomit	• Allergic reactions as anaphylactic shock or located rash • Heart palpitations • Dizziness • Muscle spasms of the neck and scapula-vertebral region • Risk of infection

Table 5. Iron therapy: Indication and side effects of enteral versus parenteral administration.

http://dx.doi.org/10.5772/intechopen.80940

Administration of IV products leads to reduced transfusion requirements for certain patients reducing the risk of posttransfusion adverse reactions.

Several iron products are available for IV administration; the most important are ferric carboxymaltose (FCM), ferric gluconate (FG), ferumoxytol, iron sucrose (IS), iron isomaltoside, and low molecular weight iron dextran (LMW ID).

Differences between these products consist in cost and the number of visits required for the administration of the total dose, namely, the time of administration and the number of doses required.

The total amount of iron required depends on the intended purpose, correcting anemia or supplementing the iron reserves.

Dose calculation is based on body weight, patient hemoglobin levels, and elemental iron/ml concentration of the product. In clinical practice, a 1000 mg dose of iron is generally enough to treat anemia. Generally, no premedication prior to IV administration is needed, except for patients with a history of asthma or drug allergies or patients with inflammatory arthritis for which 125 mg of methylprednisolone before iron administration is recommended [64].

Generally, antihistamines are not used in preventing side effects [65–67].

Administration and dosing of various iron products:

LMW Fe Dextran: It can be given in a single dose of 1000 mg in 250 ml of saline, 1 hour infusion, or multiple doses of 2 ml, i.e., 100 mg elemental Fe (2 ml ampoule, 50 mg Fe/ml).

If single dose is preferred, a test dose of 0.5 ml is administered in 30 seconds prior to the infusion.

Ferric gluconate (Ferrlecit): It is administered in a 10–15 ml dose, the equivalent of 125–187.5 mg (1 ampoule contains 12.5 mg of elemental Fe/ml). In patients with drug allergies, it is recommended to administer a test dose prior to infusion. Each dose can be given by bolus or infusion of 20–30 minutes.

Fe sucrose (Venofer): Multiple infusions with a maximum dose of 10–15 ml, equivalent to 200–300 mg of elemental Fe (ampoule 20 mg/ml), are administered. It is recommended to administer a 1.25 ml test dose (25 mg IV, administered slowly to patients with drug allergies).

Ferumoxytol: It consists of superparamagnetic iron oxide nanoparticles coated with a low molecular weight semisynthetic carbohydrate. It is administered at a dose of 17 ml, the equivalent of 510 mg elemental Fe (ampoule 30 mg/ml), with a 15 minute infusion.

Ferumoxytol may interfere with magnetic resonance imagery (MRI), which can lead to errors in interpreting the results.

Ferric carboxymaltose (Ferinject): It is used in 20 ml dose, equivalent to 1000 mg of elemental iron (the vial contains 50 mg/ml, the maximum dose being 20 mg Fe/kg body weight).

Doses are given in a 15 minute infusion. It is efficient and safe [68–71]. It can sometimes cause hypophosphatemia.

Iron isomaltoside (Monofer): It has a matrix structure where lean iron is slowly removed, allowing administration of 20 mg/kg infusion at 15 minutes; the ampoule is 100 mg/ml. It does not require a test dose. Efficacy has been demonstrated in inflammatory bowel disease, chronic renal disease, heart surgery, and chemotherapy-induced anemia [72–76].

Side effects of IV iron products:

The most common side effects consist in allergic reactions, sometimes anaphylactic shock. However, these reactions are extremely rare and often overestimated.

Patients with inflammatory arthritis (rheumatoid arthritis) may experience an exacerbation of symptoms during iron infusion, which can be prevented by administering 125 mg of methylprednisolone.

Reducing the risk of allergic reactions can be achieved through the following measures:

- Avoidance of administration of parenteral iron products to patients known for hypersensitivity reactions in the past.
- Non-premedicating patients without asthma or allergic reactions.
- Preventing the exacerbation of the symptoms of inflammatory arthritis patients by administering methylprednisolone.
- Stopping the infusion if symptoms occur.

Nonallergic reactions may occur, which include located rash, heart palpitations, dizziness, muscle spasms of the neck, scapula-vertebral region, etc.

The risk of infection may be increased because iron acts as a growth factor for bacteria. This is supported by some authors but denied by others [77, 78].

9.3. Monitoring and evaluating response to treatment

Monitoring the response to iron therapy depends on the severity of anemia and on the way of iron administration. For patients treated with oral products, reassessment is done after 2 weeks of treatment by checking Hb levels and reticulocytes. For parenteral treatment, reevaluation is done after 4–8 weeks. Iron treatment is continued until ferritin and transferrin return to normal. There are some either clinical or laboratory criteria used to monitor the efficacy of treatment with iron.

Amelioration of asthenia and installation of a well-being state in the first days of treatment besides the increased level of hemoglobin within 1–2 weeks of treatment seem to be the most important parameters related to iron-deficiency correction. In patients with severe anemia, a modest reticulocytic crisis occurs within 7–10 days after the initiation of treatment. In those with mild anemia, this reticulocytosis is not encountered.

10. Evolution and prognosis

After iron treatment, erythropoiesis with reticulocytosis efficiency occurs after 1–2 weeks of treatment, followed by an increase in hemoglobin levels. This increase (the so-called reticulocyte crisis) is not as expressed as in vitamin B12 or folic acid anemia treatment in megaloblastic anemia. With treatment, anemia is corrected in about 1–2 months, but for replenishing the iron reserves, it is necessary to continue for about 4–6 months of treatment.

Prognosis of patients with IDA depends mainly on the underlying condition that caused iron deficiency and on the cardiovascular status of patients.

Failure to respond to treatment with iron may occur in several circumstances, the more frequent observed being:

- Reduced patient compliance and treatment interruptions.
- Some conditions responsible for malabsorption in case of oral iron products.
- Excessive bleeding where oral products cannot compensate for blood loss
- Association of more types of anemia.
- Association with inflammatory disease blocking iron balance regulation.

Celiac disease and *Helicobacter pylori* infection may reduce the absorption of iron, thus being a frequent cause of failure to oral iron treatment.

An important part of fighting iron-deficiency anemia is treating its underlying cause.

Red blood cell transfusion is not generally required in iron-deficiency anemia, but in severe cases such as symptomatic patients associating cardiac pathology, transfusion is required in order to ameliorate symptoms until iron deficits are corrected.

11. Conclusion

Multiple factors can contribute to iron imbalance in the human organism. Reduced absorption, increased losses, and/or increased requirements are the main mechanisms resulting in iron deficiency. Often such factors can coexist requiring a complex management of the consequent anemia. Iron therapy should be individualized by patient's characteristics. Treatment of underlying conditions is an important step toward reducing iron-deficiency-anemia-associated morbidity.

Conflict of interest

All authors have read and approved this version of the book chapter, and due care has been taken to ensure the integrity of the work. No part of this work has been published or submitted elsewhere. No financial conflict of interest exists in the submission of this manuscript.

Author details

Claudia Burz[1,2]*, Andrei Cismaru[1,3], Vlad Pop[3] and Anca Bojan[4]

*Address all correspondence to: cburz@yahoo.fr

1 "Prof. Dr. Ion Chiricuţă" Oncology Institute, Cluj-Napoca, Cluj, Romania

2 "Iuliu Hatieganu" University of Medicine and Pharmacy, Department of Immunology and Allergology, Cluj-Napoca, Cluj, Romania

3 "Iuliu Hatieganu" University of Medicine and Pharmacy, Cluj-Napoca, Cluj, Romania

4 "Iuliu Hatieganu" University of Medicine and Pharmacy, Department of Hematology, Cluj-Napoca, Cluj, Romania

References

[1] Taylor RB. Family Medicine: Principles and Practice. 4th ed. New York; London: Springer-Verlag; 1994

[2] Thein M, Ershler WB, Artz AS, Tecson J, Robinson BE, Rothstein G, et al. Diminished quality of life and physical function in community-dwelling elderly with anemia. Medicine. 2009;**88**(2):107-114

[3] Nordenberg D, Yip R, Binkin NJ. The effect of cigarette smoking on hemoglobin levels and anemia screening. Journal of the American Medical Association. 1990;**264**(12):1556-1559

[4] Hurtado AMC, Delgado E. Influence of Anoxemia on the Hemopoietic activity. Archives of Internal Medicine. 1945;**75**(5):284-323

[5] Mehta A. Iron deficiency anemia. BMJ Best Practice. 2017

[6] Organization WH. Haemoglobin concentrations for the diagnosis of anaemia and assessment of severity. 2011:6

[7] Organization WH. Iron deficiency anaemia: Assessment, prevention and control. A Guide for Programme Managers. 2001

[8] Organization WH. WHO Global Database on Anaemia. In: Bruno de Benoist EM, editor. Worldwide prevalence of anaemia 1993-2005; 2008. p. 40

[9] Andrea U, Steinbicker MUM. Out of balance—Systemic Iron homeostasis in Iron-related disorders. Nutrients. 2013;**5**(8):3034-3061

[10] Abbaspour N, Hurrell R, Kelishadi R. Review on iron and its importance for human health. Journal of Research in Medical Sciences: The Official Journal of Isfahan University of Medical Sciences. 2014;**19**(2):164-174

[11] Ems T, Huecker MR. Biochemistry. Treasure Island (FL): Iron Absorption. StatPearls; 2018

[12] Betesh AL, Santa Ana CA, Cole JA, Fordtran JS. Is achlorhydria a cause of iron deficiency anemia? The American Journal of Clinical Nutrition. 2015;**102**(1):9-19

[13] Munoz LM, Lonnerdal B, Keen CL, Dewey KG. Coffee consumption as a factor in iron deficiency anemia among pregnant women and their infants in Costa Rica. The American Journal of Clinical Nutrition. 1988;**48**(3):645-651

[14] Monzon H, Forne M, Esteve M, Rosinach M, Loras C, Espinos JC, et al. Helicobacter pylori infection as a cause of iron deficiency anaemia of unknown origin. World Journal of Gastroenterology. 2013;**19**(26):4166-4171

[15] Geissler C, Singh M. Iron, meat and health. Nutrients. 2011;**3**(3):283-316

[16] Domellof M, Georgieff MK. Postdischarge Iron requirements of the preterm infant. The Journal of Pediatrics. 2015;**167**(4 Suppl):S31-S35

[17] Shinar S, Skornick-Rapaport A, Maslovitz S. Iron supplementation in twin pregnancy - the benefit of doubling the Iron dose in Iron deficient pregnant women: A randomized controlled trial. Twin Research and Human Genetics: The Official Journal of the International Society for Twin Studies. 2017;**20**(5):419-424

[18] Rufer A, Criblez D, Wuillemin WA. Iron-deficiency anemia and gastrointestinal bleeding. Therapeutische Umschau Revue therapeutique. 2006;**63**(5):339-343

[19] Pauwelyn KA, Verhamme M. Large hiatal hernia and iron deficiency anaemia: Clinico-endoscopical findings. Acta Clinica Belgica. 2005;**60**(4):166-172

[20] Annibale B, Capurso G, Chistolini A, D'Ambra G, DiGiulio E, Monarca B, et al. Gastrointestinal causes of refractory iron deficiency anemia in patients without gastrointestinal symptoms. The American Journal of Medicine. 2001;**111**(6):439-445

[21] Gasche C, Lomer MC, Cavill I, Weiss G. Iron, anaemia, and inflammatory bowel diseases. Gut. 2004;**53**(8):1190-1197

[22] Kluiber RM, Wolff BG. Evaluation of anemia caused by hemorrhoidal bleeding. Diseases of the Colon and Rectum. 1994;**37**(10):1006-1007

[23] Ludwig H, Evstatiev R, Kornek G, Aapro M, Bauernhofer T, Buxhofer-Ausch V, et al. Iron metabolism and iron supplementation in cancer patients. Wiener Klinische Wochenschrift. 2015;**127**(23-24):907-919

[24] Isanaka S, Mugusi F, Urassa W, Willett WC, Bosch RJ, Villamor E, et al. Iron deficiency and anemia predict mortality in patients with tuberculosis. The Journal of Nutrition. 2012;**142**(2):350-357

[25] Palacios S. The management of iron deficiency in menometrorrhagia. Gynecological Endocrinology: The Official Journal of the International Society of Gynecological Endocrinology. 2011;**27**(1 Suppl):1126-1130

[26] Simms-Stewart D, Fletcher H. Counselling patients with uterine fibroids: A review of the management and complications. Obstetrics and Gynecology International. 2012; **2012**:539365

[27] Jimenez K, Kulnigg-Dabsch S, Gasche C. Management of Iron Deficiency Anemia. Gastroenterology & Hepatology. 2015;**11**(4):241-250

[28] Ziegelstein RC, Rayburn BK, Quinlan DM. Grossly neglected hematuria: A rare cause of iron-deficiency anemia. The American Journal of Medicine. 1991;**90**(6):764-765

[29] Chikazawa S, Hoshi F, Kanai K. Repeated phlebotomies decrease body iron storage in adult dogs. The Journal of Veterinary Medical Science. 2017;**79**(10):1652-1655

[30] Aoun M, Karam R, Sleilaty G, Antoun L, Ammar W. Iron deficiency across chronic kidney disease stages: Is there a reverse gender pattern? PLoS One. 2018;**13**(1):e0191541

[31] Turgeon ML. Clinical Hematology: Theory and Procedures. 4th ed. Philadelphia, Pa., London: Lippincott Williams & Wilkins; 2005

[32] Steele TM, Frazer DM, Anderson GJ. Systemic regulation of intestinal iron absorption. IUBMB Life. 2005;**57**(7):499-503

[33] Johnson-Wimbley TD, Graham DY. Diagnosis and management of iron deficiency anemia in the 21st century. Therapeutic Advances in Gastroenterology. 2011;**4**(3):177-184

[34] Beard JL, Dawson H, Pinero DJ. Iron metabolism: A comprehensive review. Nutrition Reviews. 1996;**54**(10):295-317

[35] Bothwell TH, Cook JD, Finch CA. Iron metabolism in man. Experimental Physiology. 1980;**65**(3):255-256

[36] Disler PB, Lynch SR, Charlton RW, Torrance JD, Bothwell TH, Walker RB, et al. The effect of tea on iron absorption. Gut. 1975;**16**(3):193-200

[37] Beaumont C, Delaby C. Recycling iron in normal and pathological states. Seminars in Hematology. 2009;**46**(4):328-338

[38] Knovich MA, Storey JA, Coffman LG, Torti SV, Torti FM. Ferritin for the clinician. Blood Reviews. 2009;**23**(3):95-104

[39] Gottlieb Y, Topaz O, Cohen LA, Yakov LD, Haber T, Morgenstern A, et al. Physiologically aged red blood cells undergo erythrophagocytosis in vivo but not in vitro. Haematologica. 2012;**97**(7):994-1002

[40] Ganz T. Systemic iron homeostasis. Physiological Reviews. 2013;**93**(4):1721-1741

[41] Waldvogel-Abramowski S, Waeber G, Gassner C, Buser A, Frey BM, Favrat B, et al. Physiology of iron metabolism. Transfusion medicine and hemotherapy: Offizielles Organ der Deutschen Gesellschaft fur Transfusionsmedizin und Immunhamatologie. 2014; **41**(3):213-221

[42] Camaschella C, Nai A. Ineffective erythropoiesis and regulation of iron status in iron loading anaemias. British Journal of Haematology. 2016;**172**(4):512-523

[43] Drakesmith H, Nemeth E, Ganz T. Ironing out Ferroportin. Cell Metabolism. 2015;**22**(5): 777-787

[44] Chung M, Chan JA, Moorthy D, Hadar N, Ratichek SJ, Concannon TW, et al. Biomarkers for Assessing and Managing Iron Deficiency Anemia in Late-Stage Chronic Kidney Disease: Future Research Needs: Identification of Future Research Needs from Comparative Effectiveness Review No 83. Rockville (MD): AHRQ Future Research Needs Papers; 2013

[45] Ozdemir N. Iron deficiency anemia from diagnosis to treatment in children. Turk pediatri arsivi. 2015;**50**(1):11-19

[46] Joosten E. Iron deficiency anemia in older adults: A review. Geriatrics & Gerontology International. 2018;**18**(3):373-379

[47] Umbreit J. Iron deficiency: A concise review. American Journal of Hematology. 2005; **78**(3):225-231

[48] Naigamwalla DZ, Webb JA, Giger U. Iron deficiency anemia. The Canadian veterinary journal = La revue veterinaire canadienne. 2012;**53**(3):250-256

[49] Liu K, Kaffes AJ. Iron deficiency anaemia: A review of diagnosis, investigation and management. European Journal of Gastroenterology and Hepatology. 2012;**24**(2):109-116

[50] De Franceschi L, Iolascon A, Taher A, Cappellini MD. Clinical management of iron deficiency anemia in adults: Systemic review on advances in diagnosis and treatment. European Journal of Internal Medicine. 2017;**42**:16-23

[51] Stein J, Hartmann F, Dignass AU. Diagnosis and management of iron deficiency anemia in patients with IBD. Nature Reviews. Gastroenterology & Hepatology. 2010;**7**(11): 599-610

[52] Nairz M, Theurl I, Wolf D, Weiss G. Iron deficiency or anemia of inflammation? : Differential diagnosis and mechanisms of anemia of inflammation. Wiener Medizinische Wochenschrift. 2016;**166**(13-14):411-423

[53] Massey AC. Microcytic anemia. Differential diagnosis and management of iron deficiency anemia. The Medical Clinics of North America. 1992;**76**(3):549-566

[54] Urrechaga E, Hoffmann JJ, Izquierdo S, Escanero JF. Differential diagnosis of microcytic anemia: The role of microcytic and hypochromic erythrocytes. International Journal of Laboratory Hematology. 2015;**37**(3):334-340

[55] Hempel EV, Bollard ER. The evidence-based evaluation of Iron deficiency Anemia. The Medical Clinics of North America. 2016;**100**(5):1065-1075

[56] Institute of Medicine. Committee on the Prevention D, Management of Iron Deficiency Anemia Among USC, Women of Childbearing A, Earl RO, Woteki CE. Iron deficiency anemia: Recommended guidelines for the prevention, detection, and management among U.S. children and women of childbearing age. Washington, D.C.: National Academy Press; 1993

[57] Grasso P. Sarcoma after intramuscular iron injection. British Medical Journal. 1973; **2**(5867):667

[58] Greenberg G. Sarcoma after intramuscular iron injection. British Medical Journal. 1976;**1**(6024):1508-1509

[59] Modepalli N, Shivakumar HN, McCrudden MT, Donnelly RF, Banga A, Murthy SN. Transdermal delivery of Iron using soluble microneedles: Dermal kinetics and safety. Journal of Pharmaceutical Sciences. 2016;**105**(3):1196-1200

[60] Auerbach M, Schrier S. Treatment of iron deficiency is getting trendy. The Lancet Haematology. 2017;**4**(11):e500-e5e1

[61] Stoffel NU. Iron absorption from oral iron supplements given on consecutive versus alternate days and as single morning doses versus twice-daily split dosing in iron-depleted women: Two open-label, randomised controlled trials. The Lancet Haematology. 2017; **4**(11):524-533

[62] Rimon E, Kagansky N, Kagansky M, Mechnick L, Mashiah T, Namir M, et al. Are we giving too much iron? Low-dose iron therapy is effective in octogenarians. The American Journal of Medicine. 2005;**118**(10):1142-1147

[63] Cook JD, Reddy MB. Effect of ascorbic acid intake on nonheme-iron absorption from a complete diet. The American Journal of Clinical Nutrition. 2001;**73**(1):93-98

[64] Auerbach M, Chaudhry M, Goldman H, Ballard H. Value of methylprednisolone in prevention of the arthralgia-myalgia syndrome associated with the total dose infusion of iron dextran: A double blind randomized trial. The Journal of Laboratory and Clinical Medicine. 1998;**131**(3):257-260

[65] Camaschella C. Iron-deficiency anemia. The New England Journal of Medicine. 2015; **372**(19):1832-1843

[66] Rampton D, Folkersen J, Fishbane S, Hedenus M, Howaldt S, Locatelli F, et al. Hypersensitivity reactions to intravenous iron: Guidance for risk minimization and management. Haematologica. 2014;**99**(11):1671-1676

[67] Bircher AJ, Auerbach M. Hypersensitivity from intravenous iron products. Immunology and Allergy Clinics of North America. 2014;**34**(3):707-723 x-xi

[68] Steinmetz T, Tschechne B, Harlin O, Klement B, Franzem M, Wamhoff J, et al. Clinical experience with ferric carboxymaltose in the treatment of cancer- and chemotherapy-associated anaemia. Annals of oncology: Official Journal of the European Society for Medical Oncology. 2013;**24**(2):475-482

[69] Bregman DB, Morris D, Koch TA, He A, Goodnough LT. Hepcidin levels predict nonresponsiveness to oral iron therapy in patients with iron deficiency anemia. American Journal of Hematology. 2013;**88**(2):97-101

[70] Van Wyck DB, Martens MG, Seid MH, Baker JB, Mangione A. Intravenous ferric carboxymaltose compared with oral iron in the treatment of postpartum anemia: A randomized controlled trial. Obstetrics and Gynecology. 2007;**110**(2 Pt 1):267-278

[71] Macdougall IC, Bock AH, Carrera F, Eckardt KU, Gaillard C, Van Wyck D, et al. FIND-CKD: A randomized trial of intravenous ferric carboxymaltose versus oral iron in patients with chronic kidney disease and iron deficiency anaemia. Nephrology, dialysis, transplantation: Official publication of the European Dialysis and Transplant Association-European Renal Association. 2014;**29**(11):2075-2084

[72] Reinisch W, Staun M, Tandon RK, Altorjay I, Thillainayagam AV, Gratzer C, et al. A randomized, open-label, non-inferiority study of intravenous iron isomaltoside 1,000 (Monofer) compared with oral iron for treatment of anemia in IBD (PROCEED). The American Journal of Gastroenterology. 2013;**108**(12):1877-1888

[73] Bhandari S, Kalra PA, Kothari J, Ambuhl PM, Christensen JH, Essaian AM, et al. A randomized, open-label trial of iron isomaltoside 1000 (Monofer(R)) compared with iron sucrose (Venofer(R)) as maintenance therapy in haemodialysis patients. Nephrology, dialysis, transplantation: Official publication of the European Dialysis and Transplant Association—European Renal Association. 2015;**30**(9):1577-1589

[74] Kalra PA, Bhandari S, Saxena S, Agarwal D, Wirtz G, Kletzmayr J, et al. A randomized trial of iron isomaltoside 1000 versus oral iron in non-dialysis-dependent chronic kidney disease patients with anaemia. Nephrology, Dialysis, Transplantation: Official Publication of the European Dialysis and Transplant Association—European Renal Association. 2016;**31**(4):646-655

[75] Birgegard G, Henry D, Glaspy J, Chopra R, Thomsen LL, Auerbach M. A randomized noninferiority trial of intravenous Iron Isomaltoside versus Oral Iron sulfate in patients with nonmyeloid malignancies and Anemia receiving chemotherapy: The PROFOUND trial. Pharmacotherapy. 2016;**36**(4):402-414

[76] Johansson PI, Rasmussen AS, Thomsen LL. Intravenous iron isomaltoside 1000 (Monofer(R)) reduces postoperative anaemia in preoperatively non-anaemic patients undergoing elective or subacute coronary artery bypass graft, valve replacement or a combination thereof: A randomized double-blind placebo-controlled clinical trial (the PROTECT trial). Vox Sanguinis. 2015;**109**(3):257-266

[77] Avni T, Bieber A, Grossman A, Green H, Leibovici L, Gafter-Gvili A. The safety of intravenous iron preparations: Systematic review and meta-analysis. Mayo Clinic Proceedings. 2015;**90**(1):12-23

[78] Marx JJ. Iron and infection: Competition between host and microbes for a precious element. Best Practice & Research. Clinical Haematology. 2002;**15**(2):411-426

Chapter 2

Iron Deficiency and Iron Deficiency Anemia in Children

Roberto Miniero, Valentina Talarico,
Maria Concetta Galati, Laura Giancotti,
Paola Saracco and Giuseppe Raiola

Additional information is available at the end of the chapter

http://dx.doi.org/10.5772/intechopen.79790

Abstract

Iron deficiency anemia is considered the most common and widespread nutritional form of anemia in childhood. Red cells are hypochromic and microcytic with low mean corpuscular volume (MCV), low mean corpuscular hemoglobin (MCH) and low reticulocyte hemoglobin content (CHr). Red blood cell distribution width (RDW) is increased. Serum iron is reduced, transferrin is increased and serum ferritin is decreased. Prematurity, decreased dietary source, malabsorption and blood loss represent the most common causes of iron deficiency. Recommended oral dose of elemental iron is 2–6 mg/kg/day; when normal hemoglobin values are reached, treatment must be generally continued for 3 months in order to replenish iron stores. Rarely intravenous therapy is required. The pediatricians and other health care providers should strive to prevent and eliminate iron deficiency and iron-deficiency anemia.

Keywords: iron deficiency, anemia, children, hypochromic microcytic anemia, prevention

1. Introduction

In children, iron represents an essential nutrient for growth and proper function of many organs and systems, mainly erythropoiesis. It must be obtained from the diet and absorbed in the upper gastrointestinal tract. When iron requirements are not met, as when the balance of iron intake, iron stores and the body's loss are insufficient to fully support the production of erythrocytes, it is referred to as iron deficiency (ID). In 30% of cases, the ID, if left untreated, evolves in iron deficiency anemia (IDA) which represents the most frequent form of anemia in childhood.

IntechOpen

© 2018 The Author(s). Licensee IntechOpen. This chapter is distributed under the terms of the Creative Commons Attribution License (http://creativecommons.org/licenses/by/3.0), which permits unrestricted use, distribution, and reproduction in any medium, provided the original work is properly cited.

2. Epidemiology

ID and IDA are among the most widespread morbid conditions in the world and represent a public health problem both in developed and developing countries. All reports agree that IDA is the most common anemia worldwide in school-age children. A recent WHO report, obtained from 200 countries, showed a significant reduction in prevalence of ID/IDA that rose from 40.2% in 1990 to 32.9% in 2010. In countries with limited resources, ID affects about two-thirds of children and adolescents; it is estimated that around 25% of preschool children suffers from IDA. In Africa, the prevalence of IDA among school-age children still ranges from 64.3 to 71%. In Europe, the overall prevalence of ID/IDA is 2–4%, with two peaks between the first and third year of life (2.3–15%) and adolescence (3.5–13% in males, 11–33% in females). ID/IDA is less than 5% in Northern and Western Europe, but it is considerably higher in Eastern Europe (9–50%). In the United States, IDA prevalence is 1.6–7.4% among pediatric population; in children 1–5 years old, the prevalence of ID is 7–8% and about one-third of them have IDA. The prevalence is higher among children 1–2 years old (13.5 and 2.7%, respectively). Although the prevalence of IDA has decreased over the past decade, data from many surveys indicate that it remains relatively high among low-income family; the prevalence of ID/IDA was 17% in 1–2 years old and 6% in 3–4 years old among Mexican American toddlers, and 12% in 1–2 years old and 5% in 3–4 years old in other low-income family [1–7].

3. Pathophysiology

The amount of iron contained in the body, in relation to the various ages, is summarized in **Table 1**. During the first year of life, total-body iron increases by 240 mg; nearly 80% of that iron is used for expanded hemoglobin production (50%) and iron stores (30%). Over this age, iron intake or stores must remain sufficient for the ongoing growth and increased red cell mass. Iron metabolism is essentially a "closed system" in which almost all metal from the hemocateresis (about 95%) is continuously recycled to meet the demands of the various compartments, especially the production of new red blood cells (RBC). Only a small part of the body iron is represented by that absorbed from the diet. In adults, less than 5% of the iron requirement for the erythropoiesis is obtained from food while in the child the iron destined for hemoglobin synthesis derives for 30% from the diet; the remainder part come from the deposits and the rework of the iron released by the hemocateresis. From the sixth month, the total body iron progressively increases (70%) to answer to the high rate

	Newborn (3.300 kg)	Children (35 kg)	Adult (75 kg)
Total content	240–250 mg	1.5–2 g	2.5 (f)–4 (m) g
Hemoglobin	132–137.5 mg (55%)	1–1.4 g (68%)	2.00–2.72 g (50–70%)
Ferritin and hemosiderin (deposit)	101–105 mg (42%)	400–500 mg (27%)	0.81–1.08 g (15–30%)
Myoglobin		60–80 mg (4%)	120–300 mg (3–5%)
Enzymes	7–7.5 mg (3%)	9.12 mg (0.6%)	18–24 mg (0.2–5%)

Table 1. Iron content in the body in newborn, child and adult.

of growth and the expansion of the erythrocyte mass. As more than 60% of the iron absorbed is destined to this function (1 kg of weight corresponds to 75 ml of blood or 9 g of hemoglobin and 30 mg of iron). It is clear that in this age, iron balance is more precarious, and possible dietary imbalances could reduce tolerance limits (delayed weaning, vegetarian diet and malabsorption).

Physiological losses are minimal (about 0.5–1 mg/day) and are mostly due to exfoliation of the mucous membranes (bile, intestine, kidneys and lungs) and of the skin. Since there are no specific mechanisms of iron excretion through the liver or kidneys, iron balance is mainly controlled at the intestinal level by modulating its absorption. A balanced diet of an adult contains about 10–15 mg of iron. The absorption of iron in the foods, which varies from 5 to 15% (up to 20% for the meal), compensates the physiological losses. In case of blood losses (menstruation or other bleeding), acute or chronic hemolytic events, or periods of increased demand, such as rapid growth, pregnancy and competitive sports activity, intestinal absorption can increase up to four times.

Regarding the developmental age, the iron requirement (LARN 2014) to be taken with the diet, after 6 months is about 7–11 mg/day which corresponds to about 0.8–1 mg of iron absorbed. Of these, around 75% are used for growth and 25% to offset the losses. In adolescent age, after the appearance of the menarche (considering that with each menstrual cycle are lost about 10–25 mg of iron), the amount to be taken with the diet rises to 13–18 mg/day [6–15].

4. Etiology

The causes of iron deficiency are numerous, but in the children, these are basically due to four causes: decreased reserves at birth, inadequate intake with the diet, reduced intestinal absorption or chronic losses of blood. **Table 2** examines all causes [1–4]. "Physiological anemia"

Decreased reserves at birth: prematurity and/or twinning, intrauterine fetus-fetal and fetus-maternal transfusions, exanguino-transfusion at birth or severe IDA in the mother, early clamping of the umbilical cord.
Inadequate intake: late weaning, incongruous diet (uncontrolled vegetarian-vegan) and/or increased needs: rapid weight-growth such as low birth weight, prematurity, adolescent development and cyanotic heart disease.
Reduced absorption: celiac disease, intestinal bowel disease, Hirschsprung disease, large intestinal resections (short bowel), use of antacids and proton pump inhibitors, excess in the diet of phytates (soy and cereals), bran, starch, calcium, polyphenols (tea and coffee), soy protein, casein and egg white, *Helicobacter pylori* infection, giardiasis and other intestinal parasites, obesity, bariatric surgery, immune deficiencies with mucosal atrophy, intestinal lymphangiectasia.
Blood loss: abundant and/or frequent menstruation, intolerance of cow's milk protein, consumption more than 500 ml/day of cow-milk, Meckel's diverticulum, esophageal varices, polyps and hemorrhoids, intestinal bowel disease, intestinal parasitosis, epistaxis, severe hematuria, prolonged use of aspirin, cortisones, nonsteroidal anti-inflammatory drugs, frequent blood sampling for diagnostic purposes (in the newborn, especially if immature, and in the small infant).
Hereditary forms (rare diseases): DMT1 deficiency, transferrin deficiency, refractory iron deficiency anemia (IRIDA).
Chronic pulmonary diseases: pulmonary hemosiderosis, cystic fibrosis, bronchopulmonary dysplasia.
Iron deficiency anemia associated with anemia of chronic diseases.

Table 2. Main causes of iron deficiency in childhood and adolescence.

develops in the postnatal period, and iron stores are sufficient to provide erythropoiesis in the first 6 months of life if there is no significant blood loss. In low birth weight infants and in babies with perinatal blood loss, the stores are exhausted earlier. The amount of iron in breast milk is at the highest level in the first month, but it decreases gradually in the subsequent periods and is reduced up to 0.3 mg/l approximately in the fifth month. Although the amount of iron received from breast milk is typically low, its absorption is considerably high (50%). Solid foods, given after the sixth month, should be rich especially in iron, zinc, phosphorus, magnesium, calcium and vitamin B6. According to the WHO data, 98% of the iron requirement in infants aged 6–23 months should be introduced by solid foods. In patients, especially in older children and adolescents, blood losses should be considered, if inadequate intake can be excluded or there is inadequate response to iron treatment.

5. Clinical presentation

Mild iron deficiency, without anemia, mostly occurs asymptomatic or can only occur with poor exercise tolerance and/or asthenia. With the worsening of iron deficiency, asthenia becomes more relevant, especially in relation to the reduced amount of myoglobin and enzymes for the oxidative phosphorylation. When anemia appears, the most significant symptom is pallor of the mucous membranes and of the skin. In about 10% of children with IDA, there is modest splenomegaly as a result of mild hemolysis. The reduction in hemoglobin is slow. The child is

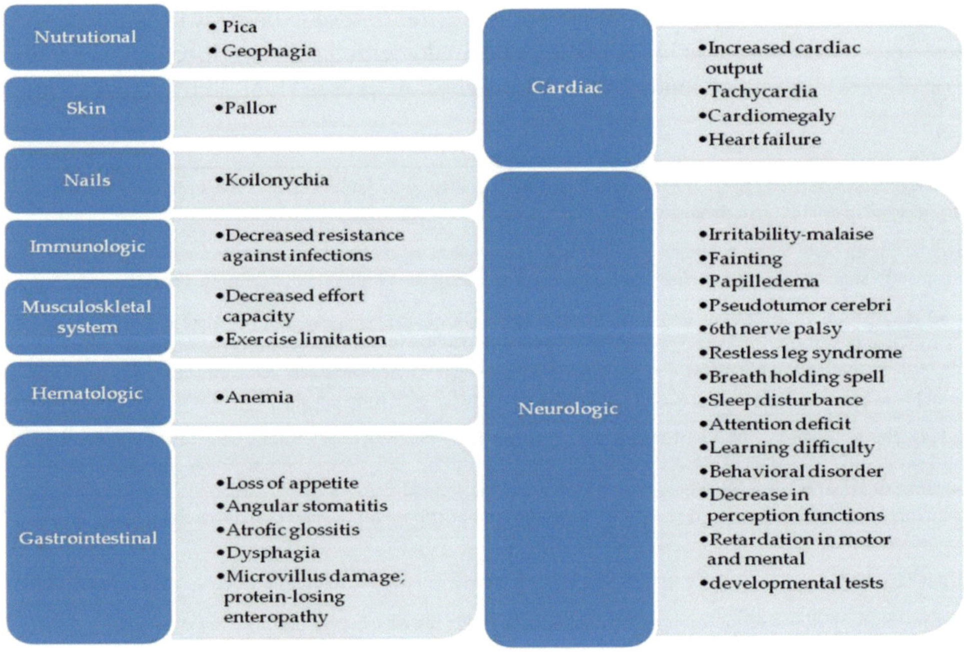

Figure 1. Manifestation and multisystem sequelae of iron deficiency.

able to compensate poor tissue oxygenation without significant clinical manifestations except for a modest tachycardia, with an increase in cardiac output and a moderate tachypnea. This mechanism is due to an increase of 2,3-diphosphoglycerate (2-3-DPG) in red blood cells, that induces a displacement to the right of the dissociation curve of the hemoglobin, allows a greater release of oxygen to the tissues.

Whereas iron plays a fundamental role in numerous metabolic processes in different organs and tissues, its deficiency is not only reflected on erythropoiesis but can also have consequences at various levels. The preschooler children may show lack of appetite, lack of desire to play and sometimes irritability; the older child can have asthenia, listlessness, headache and reduced school performance. Recent literature highlights the association between chronic iron deficiency and possible compromise of the central nervous system, with intellectual, attention, memory, learning, fine motor skills and verbal fluency deficits. Some studies have shown an association between iron deficiency and increased risk of developing stroke, idiopathic intracranial hypertension, cranial nerve paralysis, sleep disorders, febrile seizures and attention deficit and hyperactivity disorder (ADHD). Iron deficiency and chronic anemia can cause glossitis, angular cheilitis, dysphagia, reduction of gastric acidity, nail dystrophy, hair fragility, amenorrhea, slowing of growth and greater susceptibility to infections. In severe forms (hardly observable in our social context), we can observe pica (ingestion of nonnutritive substances) and/or geophagy (ingestion of earth or mud) [1–4, 7, 8, 14–20] (**Figure 1**).

6. Laboratory findings

Table 3 shows the normal values of the erythrocyte parameters in relation to age. In IDA hemoglobin, red blood cells and hematocrit are below two standard deviation (SD) respect normal value according to the age, gender and race. Typically, peripheral blood smear shows hypochromic (pale) and microcytic erythrocytes with variable size and shape (anisopoikilocytosis). Subtle change in morphologic features may be observed before than overt anemia occurs, as manifestation of iron-deficient erythropoiesis. Change of red cell distribution, evaluated by red cell distribution width (RDW) and hemoglobin distribution (HDS) usually are present before overt microcytosis (reduction of MCV) and hypochromia (reduction of MCH and MCHC) are observed. The values of the iron system parameters (serum iron, transferrin, total iron binding capacity and ferritin) undergo variations due to age and are summarized in **Table 4**. In ID/IDA, serum iron is reduced (less than 50 μg/dl), and serum transferrin is increased. Transferrin saturation index below 16% is considered very sensitive for IDA. Measurement of serum ferritin is currently the laboratory test recommended for diagnosing iron deficiency. In the absence of an associated disease, a low value is an early and highly specific indicator of ID. The WHO criteria proposed to define depleted iron storages are 12 μg/l for children under 5 years and 15 μg/l for those over 5 years. However, because ferritin is an acute-phase reactive protein, it may be elevated by infection, acute and chronic inflammatory disorders, malignant disease, liver disease and starvation. In particular, in case of infection or inflammation the cut-off for serum ferritin for diagnosis of IDA is elevated

Age	Hb (g/dl)		Ht (%)		GR (10^2/l)		MCV (fl)		MCH (pg)		MCHC (g/dl)	
	Mean	−2SD	Mean	−2SD	Mean	−2SD	Mean	−2SD	Mean	−2SD	Mean	−2SD
Bird	16.5	13.5	51	42	4.7	3.9	108	98	34	31	33	30
1–3 days	18.5	14.5	56	45	5.3	4.0	108	95	34	31	33	29
1 week	17.5	13.5	54	42	5.1	3.9	107	88	34	28	33	28
2 weeks	16.5	12.5	51	39	4.9	3.6	105	86	34	28	33	28
1 month	14.0	10.0	43	31	4.2	3.0	104	85	34	28	33	29
2 months	11.5	9.0	35	28	3.8	2.7	96	77	30	26	33	29
3–6 months	11.5	9.5	35	29	3.8	3.1	91	74	30	25	33	30
0.5–2 years	12.0	10.5	36	33	4.5	3.7	78	70	27	23	33	30
2–6 years	12.5	11.5	37	34	4.6	3.9	81	75	27	24	34	31
6–12 years	13.5	11.5	40	35	4.6	4.0	86	77	29	25	34	31
2–18 years												
Female	14.0	12.0	41	36	4.6	4.1	90	78	30	25	34	31
Male	14.5	13.0	43	37	4.9	4.5	88	78	30	25	34	31
Adults												
Female	14.0	12.0	41	36	4.6	4.0	90	80	30	26	34	31
Male	15.5	13.5	47	41	5.2	4.5	90	80	30	26	34	31

Table 3. Normal erythrocyte parameters in developmental age.

to 30–50 μg/l. Combining the evaluation of the levels of c-reactive protein (CRP) is required to rule out an inflammation. In children, serum soluble transferrin receptor (sTfR) has been reported to be a sensitive indicator of iron deficiency and is appeared to be relatively less influenced by inflammation than ferritin. Unfortunately, reference values of these parameters in children are not available and not all laboratories may perform it. So far, in routine practice, evaluation of sTfR is not needed for a diagnosis of IDA. Reticulocyte hemoglobin (CHr) is another parameter useful for the diagnosis of ID. Values less than 27.5 pg are considered very sensitive and specific for IDA (83 and 72%, respectively). Measurement of red blood cell protoporphyrin IX and zinc protoporphyrin (ZPP), that are increased in IDA, provides another parameter that may help in the diagnosis. The combination of red blood cell parameters with serum ferritin and transferrin saturation index still remains the common approach to investigate anemia for the diagnosis of IDA. Serum hepcidin is a promising novel biomarker for the diagnosis of iron disorders. It is decreased in ID, and its levels may become undetectable in severe cases of IDA. As this marker is influenced by inflammation, renal and liver function, these conditions should be assessed. In the future, when commercial test for measurement of urinary or serum hepcidin will be available, these parameters might be useful in differential diagnosis. Thrombocytosis (platelets count between 500,000 and 700,000 mcL) occurs frequently. In severe forms of IDA may be present a low grade of hemolysis due to the rigidity

Age	Male	Female
Ferritin	**ng/ml**	**ng/ml**
1–30 days	6–400	6–515
1–6 days	6–410	6–340
7–12 months	6–80	6–45
1–5 years	6–24	6–24
6–9 years	10–55	10–55
10–14 years	23–70	6–40
14–19 years	23–70	6–40
Serum iron	**μg/dl**	**μg/dl**
1–5 years	22–136	22–136
6–9 years	39–136	39–136
10–14 years	28–134	45–145
14–19 years	34–162	28–184
TIBC	**μg/dl**	**μg/dl**
1–5 years	268–441	268–441
6–9 years	240–508	240–508
10–14 years	302–508	318–575
14–19 years	290–570	302–564
Transferrin	**mg/dl**	**mg/dl**
1–30 days	97–205	92–208
1–6 months	106–325	128–309
7–12 months	178–357	145–364
1–3 years	196–365	149–382
4–6 years	202–350	174–399
7–9 years	149–353	186–368
10–12 years	173–380	185–377
13–15 years	171–374	193–391
16–18 years	194–348	181–416

Table 4. Values of serum ferritin, serum iron, total iron binding capacity (TIBC) and transferrin in pediatric age (ranging from 2.5 to 97.5 percentiles).

of red cell membrane, than mild increase of hemolysis markers may be observed. Bone marrow examination is no longer performed in the work-up for IDA for assessing iron stores. However, as diagnosis of iron deficiency is somewhat complex, the use of several combined indicators seems to provide the best assessment of iron status.

Iron deficiency develops in three steps. The first one is iron depletion or prelatent stage. Iron stores are lowered or absent (serum ferritin is reduced below normal cut-off) while other parameters are unchanged. In this stage, erythropoiesis is still normal. The second stage is defined as latent stage or deficiency. Iron supply for erythropoiesis became reduced; serum iron transferrin saturation are reduced as well as CHr; StfRs increases. The third stage overt IDA is characterized by a progressive impairment of erythropoiesis and modifications of hematological parameters [1–4, 8, 9, 20–32].

At the end of this process appears the hypochromic microcytic anemia characterized by:

- Reduction of Hb, RBC number and hematocrit
- Reduction of MCV, MCH and MCHC
- Hypochromic cells with a tendency to microcytosis
- Increase of RDW > 15%
- Reduction of CHr <27.5 pg
- Reduction of serum iron <30 mg/dl; increase of total serum transferrin o of TIBC, >350 mg/dl; reduction of IS <16%; reduction of serum ferritin <10–12 ng/ml
- Increase of sTfR a 10–14 mg/l
- Reduction of reticulocyte (inconstant)
- Increase of zinc protoporphyrin > 60–80 μmol/mol-heme*
- Increase of free erythrocyte protoporphyrin (FEP) > 10 mg/dl*
- Increase of platelets count (inconstant) between 600,000–1000,000 mcL
- Rarely modest hemolysis

Parameters	Iron deficiency anemia	Hetherozygous thalassimia	Anemia of chronic diseases
MCV	Reduced	Reduced	Normal
MCH	Reduced	Reduced	Reduced
MCHC	Reduced	Normal	Reduced
RDW	Increased	Normal	Normal
Ferritin	Reduced	Normal or increased	Reduced-normal-increased
Serum iron	Reduced	Normal	Reduced
Transferrin	Increased	Normal	Reduced
Serum transferrin receptor	Increased	Increased	Normal
Tranferrin saturation index	Reduced	Normale or increased	Normal
Others	Response to iron treatment	HBA_2 concentration	No response to iron treatment

Table 5. Differential diagnosis of microcytic anemia.

In the diagnostic evaluation of IDA, a correct differential diagnosis must always be made with the other forms of microcytic-hypochromic anemia, such as thalassemia and anemia of chronic diseases (**Table 5**).

7. Treatment

Despite ID/IDA are well-known medical issues, this topic is not noticed adequately, and the literature contains only few publications related to iron treatment recommendations; this resulting in part from the lack of contemporary scientific literature regarding evidence-based treatment of IDA. The therapeutic approach of ID/IDA is widely variable and often suboptimal as often pediatricians administer inadequate daily doses of iron or inappropriate iron salt formulations or too short iron replacement [38]. The principles of ID/IDA management are based on some cornerstones: confirm the diagnosis, recognition and whenever possible, management of the underlying cause(s), provide adequate iron therapy, either orally or parenterally, and finally confirm the success of the treatment (correction of the hemoglobin levels and finally replenishment of body iron storage). If diet intake is inadequate, the first step is correction of the nutritional iron intake. In cases of ID or of IDA with good levels of hemoglobin, this approach may be sufficient to correct iron depletion. Usually, dietary counseling and oral iron therapy are combined.

Limited high-quality evidence supports the management of iron deficiency anemia. Oral iron replacement is preferred primarily because it is economical and has few side effects. Oral iron supplement is the treatment of choice by selecting the most appropriate compound, whereas parenteral route of administration is recommended only for selected patients. Iron-containing oral preparations currently available in the market are innumerous, with a variety of pharmaceutical forms including liquid preparations as guts, elixir, syrups, pills and effervescent tablets. Unfortunately, oral iron formulations are known to be far from ideal, mainly because of absorption and tolerability; also the palatability of the liquid preparation is often a real problem for children. Stain of teeth may occur if not thoroughly cleaned. Their chemistry is also heterogeneous, including either divalent (Fe^{2+}, or ferrous) or trivalent (Fe^{3+}, or ferric) iron, in form of iron salts or their complex-forming substrate iron. Treatment must correct hemoglobin levels and then gradually replenish iron stores. The time required varies from 3 to 6 months after the anemia is relieved. If the treatment is not continued, relapse is common. What really matter in different oral iron preparations is the content of elemental iron absorption. As a general rule, oral iron preparations do not contain more than 30% of elemental iron, but a source of confusion is represented by the fact that such proportion can vary by manufacturer, as well as in different countries. Ferrous formulations are recommended by international literature, scientific societies and international agencies as the preparations that are more effective. Ferric iron is poorly and ineffectively absorbed. The ferrous sulfate was first introduced by the French physician Pierre Blaud in the last half of 1800 and still remains the mainstay of treatment for adults as reasonable well absorbed, effective and inexpensive. Unfortunately, the tolerability of this salt is poor, making it unacceptable for many patients. Therefore, many other effective ferrous salts have been offered as ferrous gluconate, ferrous ascorbate, ferrous lactate, ferrous succinate, ferrous fumarate and ferrous glycine sulfate.

No one compound seems better than the others. Recent studies showed that ferrous bisglycinate chelate and ferrous bisglycinate chelate plus alginic acid have a good absorption at reduced doses (25–40%) in comparison with ferrous sulfate and an optimal tolerance. Unfortunately iron formulations, especially in older children and adolescent, may induce gastrointestinal discomfort mainly represented by including metallic taste, vomiting, heartburn, epigastric and abdominal pain, nausea, flatulence, dyspepsia, constipation and diarrhea. Likely due to the oxidative properties of iron on the gastrointestinal mucosa, these problems occur frequently, especially when iron is taken fasting. The stool often may turn black, which is not harmful, and treatment does not have to be interrupted. When side effects occur, iron can be taken with meals. Alternatively, smaller doses could be taken between meals. Ascorbic acid may improve the bioavailability of iron salts, but it increases the frequency of side effects. As the treatment is long, a good compliance is required for the success of the therapy. For this reason, the best tolerated preparation and schedule must be tailored for each patient in order to encourage compliance.

Standard dose is 2–6 mg/kg/day in terms of elemental iron, in 2–3 divided doses up to a maximum of 150–200 mg daily. It may be recommended to start treatment with low dose increasing day by day to full doses during 7–10 days. However, the optimum frequency of daily doses is uncertain. Single dose daily is well tolerated and effective when compared to divided dose, especially in children less than 2 years. Administration on empty stomach before sleeping seems to be more effective as decreased gastrointestinal motility of sleep enhance absorption. The absorptive capacity of iron in the duodenum is near complete saturated with about 25 mg of iron. It is conceivable that the treatment on 25 mg/day saturates the intestinal absorption capacity so that the next day doses are much less absorbed. It is interesting that in children with gastrointestinal side effects, iron administration once every other day or twice a week might be more effective than daily doses and might reduce gastrointestinal discomfort.

When patients do not tolerate full doses, a less iron dose may be administrated, but in this case, it is necessary to treat longer.

As gastrointestinal discomforts are more frequent when the stomach is empty, patients prefer to take iron immediately after or even with meal. Also, if it is clear that in this way the absorption is reduced to 30%, the better compliance to iron treatment may be preferred than a better absorbent. However, it is important to inform the patients that in this case some foods may influence iron absorption: orange juice, meat, poultry and fish enhance absorption while food high in phytates, phosphates or tannates (e.g., cereals, beans, soys, tea and milk) reduce it. The ensuing reduction of adherence, in combination with the need of prolonged treatment, results in undertreatment significant proportion of IDA patients in daily clinical practice. There has been an increasing awareness of a previously overlooked potentially negative effect of oral iron, that is, the change in gut microbiome. In the absence of ongoing blood loss or intestinal malabsorption response to iron treatment is rapid. So far, within 24 h, the child feels better, shows less irritability and an increased appetite. A peak of reticulocytes may observe at 5–7 days but routinely this re-evaluation is not performed in children to avoid discomfort. The hemoglobin measured after a month of treatment shows an increase of 1–2 g/dl. Since IDA has been treated and hemoglobin concentrations are healthy, full blood count and markers of iron status should be measured during the subsequent 6–12 months.

Treatment failure is common due to poor medication adherence, adverse effects related to excessive dosing and lack of evidence-based management guidelines. If after a month of treatment the anemia, in otherwise healthy individual, does not respond, the causes of the iron deficiency anemia must be carefully reevaluated. It is important to analyze the duration of therapy, ongoing blood loss, high gastric pH due to assumption of antacid, histamine-2 blocker, gastric acid pump inhibitor, deficit of Vitamin B12, folic acid, zinc, or hypothyroidism, a coexistent disease that interferes with iron absorption (chronic inflammation and inflammatory bowel disease or neoplasia). Finally, an incorrect diagnosis of the microcytic anemia, as thalassemia, sideroblastic anemia or genetic IRIDA as well as patients with elevated hepcidin levels driven by inflammation, must be ruled out. Unfortunately, many patients are often lost to follow-up [1–3, 22–24].

Considering the risk of adverse reaction, parenteral iron therapy should be reserved for selected patients with severe gastrointestinal absorption disorders including inflammatory bowel disease or short bowel syndrome, or when a rapid replacement of iron is required or an absolute intolerance to oral administration is demonstrated. There not indications of parenteral iron treatment for pediatric patients with celiac disease in gluten-free diet as they can absorb oral iron salt preparations with good clinical results. Of interest the observation that ferrous bisglycinate chelate is well absorbed also in patients with overt celiac disease (personal data-in press Minerva Pediatrica 2018).

The benefits of new generation parenteral formulations are greater than their risks, if adequate measures are taken to ensure the early detection and effective management of allergic reactions. Iron preparations should only be given in a protected environment, where resuscitation facilities are available in order to treat immediately. The practice of first giving the patient a small test dose is not a reliable way to predict how the patient will respond when the full dose is given. A test dose is therefore no longer recommended but instead caution is warranted with every dose of intravenous iron that is given, even if previous administrations have been well tolerated. Various iron formulations for intravenous use are now available but the approval of the products may differ in different countries. The first parenteral iron formulation was a high molecular weight iron dextran. However, intramuscular injection of iron dextran is discouraged because it is painful, produce long-standing skin discoloration, and it may be a potential risk of developing a rhabdomyosarcoma or fibrosarcoma. Intravenous administration is no longer available due to its relatively high incidence of hypersensitivity reactions. Low-molecular weight iron dextran, introduced in the 1990s is less likely to cause such reactions but the use in now is limited as formulations with improved safety profile have been licensed. Fe-gluconate (Ferlixit®) is less dangerous but is containing benzilic acid that may cause seizure in infant less than 3 years. Fe-sucrose (Venofer®) is much more expensive but represents today the best product for children considering the low risk if reacted. Finally, new and promising preparations are now under investigation but at the moment they are not approved for pediatrics: Fe-carboxymaltose (Ferrinject®), Fe-isomaltoside (Monofer®) and Ferumoxytol (Ferraheme®). Severe hypersensitivity reactions with these preparations are exceptional. Simple recommendations to minimize the risk include slow administration with careful patient monitoring during and after treatment, an adequate clinical environment with trained staff and the avoidance of antihistamine premedication. Iron sucrose and sodium ferric gluconate are approved for both adults and children, but typically require multiple doses to achieve adequate iron replacement. For the ferric carboxymaltose, the recommended infusion time is only 15 min and is administrated once a week. It is approved in Europe and in the US for adults, not yet approved for pediatrics.

Red cell transfusion should be reserved to severe anemia, less than 5 g/dl of hemoglobin, requiring rapid correction as in children with cardiac dysfunction.

The total amount of parenteral iron to be administered may be calculated according to the following formula:

$$\text{Weight (kg)} \times \text{volemia (80 ml/kg)} \times 3.4^{*} \times \text{g (normal Hb for age} - \text{patient Hb)} \times 1.5^{**}$$

* 1 g of Hb alloy 3.4 mg of iron, ** correction to replenish stocks

The total dose should be divided into several administrations (initially every 2–3 days then every 1–2 weeks) to be given in a slow infusion (recommended in 1–4 h, the single dose should not exceed 5 mg/kg) [1–4, 31–40].

8. Prevention

In preterm infants (born at less than 37 weeks' gestation) the prevention of ID/IDA with the administration of iron is well-established practice, even if there is no clear evidence of benefits on long-term outcomes such as growth and neurobehavioral development. Infants who are exclusively breastfed should receive 1–3 mg/kg/day of elemental iron supplementation from 1–12 months of age, except for those who have had multiple blood transfusions; 1 mg/kg/day supplementation if using iron-fortified formula. For healthy full-term infants exclusively breastfed infants, the AAP recommends 1 mg/kg/day of iron supplementation at 4 months of age until appropriate iron-containing foods are introduced. WHO recommended daily iron supplementation with 60 mg of elemental iron to prevent iron deficiency in menstruating adolescent girls where the prevalence of anemia is about 20%.

According to the American Academy of Pediatrics, the prevention of iron deficiency is an important issue of public health and the universal screening, between 12 and 18 months, is useful to assess the possible risk factors [41–45].

9. Conclusion

Prevention and early diagnosis of ID and IDA in childhood are important to ensure normal growth and performance and to avoid possible damage on neurocognitive and behavioral development. Diagnostics are generally relatively easy and are based on the evaluation of a few simple hematological and biochemical parameters. Treatment may have some difficulty regarding patient's compliance. So important is the role of the pediatrician in approaching the problem of iron deficiency in every phase of the intervention, from prevention, diagnosis and treatment.

Conflict of interest

The authors declares no conflict of interest.

Author details

Roberto Miniero[1*], Valentina Talarico[1], Maria Concetta Galati[2], Laura Giancotti[1], Paola Saracco[3] and Giuseppe Raiola[1]

*Address all correspondence to: roberto.miniero@unicz.it

1 Department of Pediatric, "Pugliese-Ciaccio" Hospital, Catanzaro, Italy

2 Department of Pediatric Onco-hematology, "Pugliese-Ciaccio" Hospital, Catanzaro, Italy

3 Department of Pediatric Hematology, Health and Science City, Turin, Italy

References

[1] Lanzkowsky P. Iron deficiency anemia. In: Lanzkowsky P, editor. Manual of Pediatric Hematology and Oncology. USA: Elsevier; 2011. pp. 38-57

[2] Anrews NC, Ullrich CK, Fleming MD. Disorders of iron metabolism and sideroblastic anemia. In: Orkin SH, Nathan DG, Ginsburg D, Look AT, Fisher DE, Lux SE, editors. Nathan and Oski' Hematology of Infancy and Childhood. Canada: Sauders Elsevier; 2009. pp. 521-570

[3] Lerner NB, Sills R. Iron deficiency anemia. In: Kliegman RM, Stanton BF, Schor NF, St. Geme GV III, Behrman RE, editors. Nelson Text of Pediatrics. 20th ed. USA, Elseviere Sauders; 2016. pp. 2323-2325

[4] Krishnamurti L. Iron deficiency anemia. In: McInerny TK, Adam HM, Campbell DE, Kamat DM, Kelleher KJ, Hoekelman RA, ExOfficio, editors. Textbook of Pediatric Care. USA: American Association of Pediatrics; 2009. pp. 2201-2209

[5] Van der Merwe LF, Eussen SR. Iron status of young children in Europe. The American Journal of Clinical Nutrition. 2017;**106**(Suppl 6):1663S-1671S

[6] Dupont C. Prévalence de la carence en fer. Archives de Pédiatrie. 2017;**24**:5S45-5S481

[7] Schneider JM, Fujii ML, Lamp CL, Lönnerdal B, Dewey KG, Zidenberg-Cherr S. Anemia, iron deficiency, and iron deficiency anemia in 12-36-mo-old children from low-income families. The Journal of Clinical Nutrition. 2005;**82**:1269-1275

[8] Bruno M, De Falco L, Iolascon A. How I diagnose non-thalassemic microcytic anemias. Seminars in Hematology. 2015;**52**:270-278

[9] Camaschella C. Iron-deficiency anemia. The New England Journal of Medicine. 2015;**372**: 1832-1843

[10] Pantopoulos K, Porwal SK, Tartakoff AM, Devireddy L. Mammalian mechanisms of iron homeostasis. Biochemistry. 2012;**51**:5705-5724

[11] Beoumont C, Karim Z. Actualité du metabolism du fer. Iron metabolism: State of art. La Revue de Médecine Interne. 2012;**34**:17-25

[12] Lönnerdal B. Development of iron homeostasis in infants and young children. The American Journal of Clinical Nutrition. 2017;**106**(Suppl 6):1575S-1580S

[13] McCarthy EK, Chaoimh N, Kenny LC, Hourihane JO, Irvine AD, Murray DM, Kiely ME. Iron status, body size, and growth in the first 2 years of life. Maternal and Child Nutrition. 2018;**14**. Epub 2017

[14] Tounian P, Chouraqui JP. Iron in nutrition. Archives de Pédiatrie. 2017;**24**:5S23-5S31

[15] Cerami C. Iron nutriture of the fetus, neonate, infant and child. Annals of Nutrition and Metabolism. 2017;**71**(Suppl.3):8-14

[16] Aly SS, Fayed HM, Ismail AM, Abdel Hakeem GL. Assessment of peripheral blood lymphocyte subsets in children with iron deficiency anemia. BMC Pediatrics. 2018; **12**(18):49

[17] Domellöf M, Braegger C, Campoy C, Colomb V, Decsi T, Fewtrell M, Hojsak I, Mihatsch W, Molgaard C, Shamir R, Turck D, van Goudoever J, ESPGHAN Committee on Nutrition. Iron requirements of infants and toddlers. Journal of Pediatric Gastroenterology and Nutrition. 2014;**58**:119-129

[18] Lazoff B. Early iron deficiency has brain and behavior effects consistent with dopaminergic dysfunction. The Journal of Nutrition. 2011;**141**:740S-746S

[19] Peirano PD, Algarin CR, Chamorro RA, Reyes SC, Duran SA, Garrido MI, Lazoff B. Sleep alterations and iron deficiency anemia in infancy. Sleep Medicine. 2010;**11**:637-642

[20] Beard J. Recent evidence from human and animal studies regarding iron status and infant development. The Journal of Nutrition. 2007;**137**:524S-530S

[21] Vendt NC, Kool P, Teesalu K, Lillemäe K, Maaroos HI, Oona M. Iron deficiency and helicobacter pylori infection in children. Acta Pediatrica. 2011;**100**:1239-1243

[22] Mahoney DH. Iron deficiency in infants and young children: Screening, prevention, clinical manifestations and diagnosis. Uptodate; 19-03-2011. www.uptodate.com

[23] Johnson-Wimbley TD, Graham DY. Diagnosis and management of iron deficiency anemia in the 21st century. Therapeutic Advances in Gastroenterology. 2011;**4**:177-184

[24] Baker RD, Greer FR. Diagnosis and prevention of iron deficiency and iron-deficiency anemia in infants and young children (0-3 years of age). Pediatrics. 2010;**126**:1040-1050

[25] Urrechaga T, Borque L, Escanero FJ. The role of automated measurement of red cell subpopulations on the sysmex XE 500 analyzer in the differential diagnosis of microcytic anemia. International Journal of Laboratory Hematology. 2011;**33**:30-36

[26] Mast AE, Blinder MA, Dietzen DJ. Reticulocytes haemoglobin content. American Journal of Hematology. 2008;**83**:307-310

[27] Ullrich C, Wu A, Armsby A, Rieber S, Wingerter S, Brugnara C, Shapiro D, Bernstein H. Screening healthy infants for iron deficiency using reticulocyte haemoglobin content. Journal of the American Medical Association. 2005;**294**:24-31

[28] Parodi E, Giraudo MT, Davitto M, Ansaldi G, Mondino A, Garbarini L, Franzil A, Mazzone R, Russo G, Ramenghi U. Reticulocyte parameters markers of early response to oral treatment in children with severe iron deficiency anemia. Journal of Pediatric Hematology/Oncology. 2012;**34**:e249-e252

[29] Urrechaga T. Red blood cell microcytosis and hypocromia in the differential diagnosis of iron deficiency and B-thalassemic trait. Journal of Pediatric Hematology/Oncology. 2009;**31**:528-534

[30] Soldin OP, Bierbower LH, Choi JJ, Thompson-Hoffman S, Soldin SJ. Serum iron, ferritin, transferrin, total iron binding capacity, hs-CRP, cholesterol and magnesium in children. New reference intervals using DADE dimension clinical chemistry system. Clinical Chimica Acta. 2004;**342**:211-217

[31] Beard JL, Murray-Kolb LE, Rosales FJ, Solomons NW, Angelilli ML. Interpretation of serum ferritin concentrations as indicators of total-body iron stores in survey population: The role of biomarkers for the acute phase response. The American Journal of Clinical Nutrition. 2006;**84**:1498-1505

[32] Thuret A. Diagnostic biologique de la carence martiale chez l'enfant. Archives de Pédiatrie. 2017;**24**:5S6-5S13

[33] Thurnham DI, Mc Cabe LD, Haldar S, Wieringa FD, Northrop-Clewes CA. Adjusting plasma ferritin concentrations to remove the effects of subclinical inflammation in the assessment of iron deficiency: A meta-analysis. The American Journal of Clinical Nutrition. 2010;**92**:546-555

[34] Daru J, Colman K, Stanworth SJ, De La Salle B, Wood EW, Pasricha SR. Serum ferritin as an indicator of iron status: What do we need to know? The American Journal of Clinical Nutrition. 2017;**106**(Suppl 6):1634S-1639S

[35] Speeckaert MM, Speeckaert R, Delanghe JR. Biological and clinical aspects of soluble transferrin receptor. Critical Reviews in Clinical laboratory Science. 2011;**47**:213-228

[36] Celi J, Samii K, Perrier A, Reny JL. Anémie ferriprive, inflammatoire ou mixte: Comment orienter le diagnostic? Revue Médicale Suisse. 2011;**7**:2018-2023

[37] Bosco C, Favrat B, Cheseaux M. Carences en vitamine B12 et fer: Du diagnostic au suivi. Revue médicale suisse. 2012;**8**:1348-1351

[38] Huang S, Yang Y, Cheng C, Chen J, Lin C. The etiology and treatment outcome of iron deficiency and iron deficiency anemia in children. Journal of Pediatric Hematology/Oncology. 2010;**32**:282-285

[39] Powers JM, Daniel CL, McCavit TL, Buchanan GR. Deficiencies in the management of iron deficiency anemia during childhood. Pediatric Blood and Cancer. 2016;**63**:743-745

[40] Clénin GE. The treatment of iron deficiency without anaemia in otherwise healthy persons. The Swiss Medical Weekly. 2017;**147**:w14434

[41] Martius C. Carence martiale sans anémie—Un sujet brûlant? Conséquences non hématologiques de la carence martiale:lesquelles sont confirmées, quand sont-elles importantes? Forum Med Suisse. 2009;**9**:294-299

[42] Guideline WHO. intermittent Iron Supplementation for Preschool and School-age Children. Geneva: World Health Organization; 2011

[43] Muñoza M, Gómez-Ramírezb S, Bhandaric S. The safety of available treatment options for iron-deficiency anemia. Expert Opinion on Drug Safety. 2018;**17**:149-159

[44] McDonagh M, Blazina I, Dana T, Cantor A, Bougatsos C. Routine Iron Supplementation and Screening for Iron Deficiency Anemia in Children Ages 6 to 24 Months: A Systematic Review to Update the U.S. Preventive Services Task Force Recommendation. Agency for Healthcare Research and Quality (US). 2015 March. Report No.: 13-05187-EF-1

[45] McDonagh MS, Blazina I, Dana T, Cantor A, Bougatsos C. Screening and routine supplementation for iron deficiency anemia: A systematic review. Pediatrics. 2015;**135**(4):723-733

Chapter 3

Effect of Iron Deficiency on the Increased Blood Divalent Metal Concentrations

Yangho Kim

Additional information is available at the end of the chapter

http://dx.doi.org/10.5772/intechopen.78958

Abstract

The apical divalent metal transporter 1 (DMT1) and the iron exporter ferroportin 1 (FPN1) are responsible for the absorption of iron and other divalent metals (manganese, lead, and cadmium). Thus, an iron-deficient diet can lead to excess absorption of manganese, lead, and cadmium, and high blood concentrations of these metals. Relative to males, females of childbearing age have higher blood concentrations of manganese because of their lower blood concentrations of ferritin. Moreover, relative to premenopausal women, menopausal women have lower blood manganese levels because their higher concentrations of ferritin. There is also a significant increase in the whole blood manganese level throughout pregnancy due to the upregulation of iron absorption at this time. Several previous studies reported a temporal relationship between iron deficiency and increased blood lead concentrations in children. However, this association does not occur in postmenarcheal or postmenopausal women because estrogen promotes bone mineralization and redistributes blood lead into the bone, overshadowing the effect of ferritin on blood lead level. Although blood cadmium concentrations are higher in females of childbearing age because of their lower ferritin concentrations, there is no association of blood cadmium and iron levels in infants and postmenopausal women.

Keywords: manganese, lead, cadmium, iron deficiency, divalent metal transporter 1, ferroportin

1. Introduction

Iron deficiency affects approximately one-third of the world's population, and is the most common nutritional deficiency [1]. Iron deficiency is most common in rapidly growing children (aged 6 months

IntechOpen

© 2018 The Author(s). Licensee IntechOpen. This chapter is distributed under the terms of the Creative Commons Attribution License (http://creativecommons.org/licenses/by/3.0), which permits unrestricted use, distribution, and reproduction in any medium, provided the original work is properly cited.

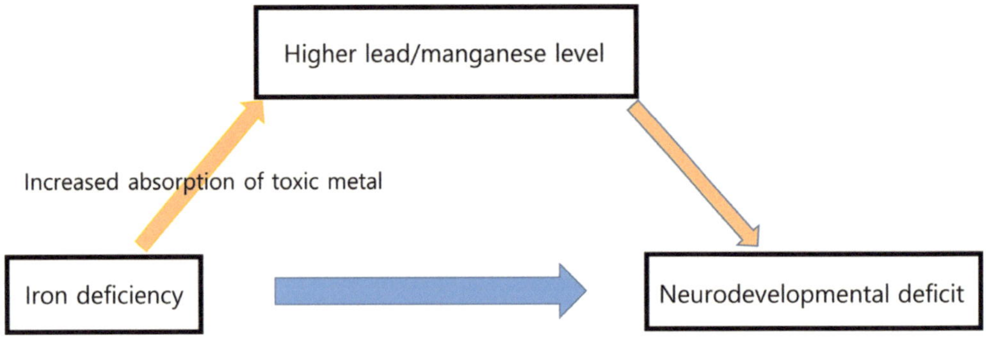

Figure 1. The direct and indirect effect of iron deficiency on neurodevelopment in children.

to 3 years) who have inadequate intake of dietary iron [2]. Iron deficiency is the only micronutrient deficiency that also has a high prevalence in virtually all developed countries [3].

Toxic metals, such as manganese, lead, and cadmium, have become ubiquitous in the developed world, and general populations are increasingly exposed to these metals. Inhalation of toxic metals is the most common route of exposure in environmental and occupational settings [4]; food intake is the major source of exposure in general populations and in children, who are more vulnerable to toxic metals absorbed through the intestine [5]. The mechanisms of iron absorption are similar to those of other divalent metals [6–11], and an iron-deficient diet can lead to excess absorption of manganese [12–14], lead [15–17], and cadmium [18–20].

The gastrointestinal absorption of these divalent metals appears to be mediated by intestinal iron transporters, such as apical divalent metal transporter 1 (DMT1), which also mediates the uptake of other divalent metals [21]. There is up-regulation of DMT1 in the presence of low iron stores [22], and this explains the increased uptake of divalent metals [13, 14] and the higher blood concentrations of these metals in iron-deficient individuals. New evidence indicates that the iron exporter ferroportin 1 (FPN1) also transports these divalent metal ions [8–11]. Thus, the major transporters responsible for the absorption of nonheme iron, apical DMT1 and the FPN1, also function in the absorption of divalent toxic metal ions.

Elevated levels of manganese, lead, and cadmium may adversely affect neurodevelopment, cognitive and motor development, and behavioral development in children [23]. Iron deficiency in children may lead to cognitive impairment, caused by the deficiency of iron itself or by the increased levels of these toxic metals (**Figure 1**). Therefore, decreased levels of iron, combined with increased levels of cadmium, manganese, or lead, have major effects on the neurodevelopment of children [24].

2. Effect of iron deficiency on blood concentrations of manganese, lead, and cadmium

2.1. Manganese

Manganese is a naturally occurring element that is abundant in the environment. It is also an essential dietary nutrient, and the body requires specific concentrations for proper function.

More specifically, at the physiological level, manganese functions in bone formation, protein and energy metabolism, and metabolic regulation; at the molecular level, it functions as a cofactor for a number of enzymes [25]. Because manganese is an essential element, homeostatic mechanisms regulate its absorption, disposition, and biliary excretion [25]. These homeostatic processes also play important roles in manganese toxicokinetics, which differ from those of nonessential toxic metals, such as lead and cadmium. Inhalation is the most common route of adult manganese exposure in environmental and occupational settings [25], whereas food is the major source of absorbed manganese in children, who are more vulnerable than adults to manganese due to higher intestinal absorption rate. Another source is the presence of a portal systemic shunt due to liver cirrhosis, which impairs the clearance of manganese through biliary excretion [25]. Blood manganese concentration appears to be related to manganese body burden on a group basis [25]. Chronic occupational exposure to manganese can cause a neurologic impairment known as "manganism," a motor disorder with some similarities to idiopathic Parkinson's disease in adults [25]. Recently, manganese excess have been reported to be associated with neurodevelopmental deficits, reduced IQ, and increased risk of behavioral problems, and attention deficit hyperactivity disorder in children [26].

Animal and human studies have demonstrated that iron deficiency markedly enhances intestinal absorption of manganese [12, 13]. DMT1 and FPN1 are responsible for the absorption of iron and other essential divalent metals, particularly manganese. Thus, an iron-deficient diet can lead to excess absorption of manganese; therefore, iron deficiency can be a risk factor for the accumulation of toxic levels of manganese in the central nervous system [27].

Previous studies have shown that iron deficiency leads to increased blood manganese concentrations in adults and children [14, 28, 29]. We recently showed that blood manganese levels are also elevated in iron-deficient infants [30]. After iron therapy, the blood manganese levels of iron-deficient infants declined significantly relative to their pretherapy levels (2.045 vs. 2.971 μg/dL), and their hemoglobin and ferritin levels increased significantly. Females of childbearing age have reduced concentrations of ferritin, and therefore increased levels of blood manganese relative to males [14, 31–33] and relative to menopausal women (who have higher levels of ferritin) [33] (**Figure 2**). Previous research reported significant increases in the whole blood manganese levels throughout pregnancy [34–38] (**Table 1**). This may be related to the enhanced absorption of manganese due to upregulation of iron absorption, particularly during the late periods of pregnancy [39], because the mechanisms of iron and manganese absorption are similar.

2.2. Lead

Lead is a widespread environmental pollutant that can damage the central nervous, peripheral nervous, renal, cardiovascular, reproductive, and hematological systems in adults [40]. Exposure to lead induces a wide range of adverse health effects in children [40], because children are more sensitive to toxic effects. Very low blood lead levels (<10 μg/dL) have been associated with reduced IQ, deficits in executive function, and attention deficit hyperactivity disorder in children [26]. The environmental exposure to lead are mainly from leaded gasoline, lead paint such as lead paint-contaminated dust and soil, water from lead pipes, and emissions due to industrial activities [40]. Thus, main route of environmental exposure to lead is inhalation or ingestion [40]. Bone lead reflects total body burden of lead. However, blood lead concentration accounts for a part of the total body burden, and it reflects a recent exposure [40].

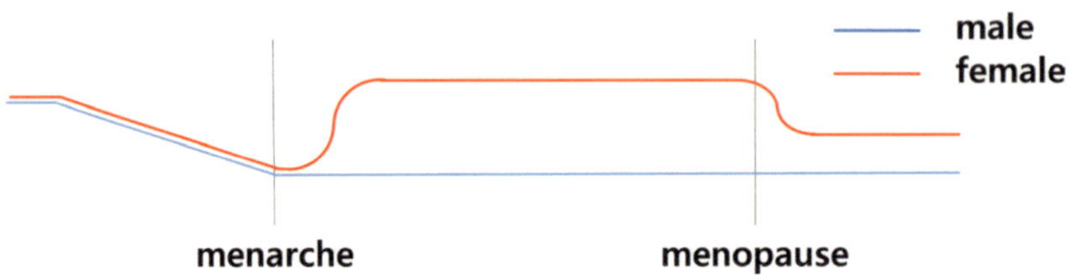

Figure 2. Changes in blood manganese levels according to sex, age, and menstrual status.

Variables	No. (n)	Study subjects and findings
Sex	(n = 2005)	Korean general population 20 y or more; KNHANES 2008/GM of blood Mn in female vs. male: 1.403 vs. 1.192 μg/dL* [14]
	(n = 297)	Canadian general population/GM of blood Mn in female vs. male: 0.750 vs. 0.675 μg/dL* [31]
	(n = 7720)	USA general population (NHANES 2010–2011)/GM of blood Mn in female vs. male: 0.99 vs. 0.87 μg/dL* [32]
Menopause	(n = 1826)	Korean general population KNHANES 2008–2009/GM of blood Mn in premenopause vs. postmenopause: 1.443 vs. 1.296 μg/dL* [33]
	(n = 66)	Sweden general population/Maternal blood median Mn during pregnancy at 3rd, vs. 2nd, vs. 1st trimester 1.26 vs. 1.04 vs. 0.85 μg/dL [34]
Pregnancy	(n = 34)	Australian general population/Maternal blood Mn during pregnancy from 10 to 20 weeks vs. 25 vs. 34 weeks; 0.82 vs. 0.94 vs. 1.26 μg/dL [35]
	(n = 290)	Canadian general population/Maternal blood GM Mn during pregnancy at 3rd, vs. 2nd, vs. 1st trimester vs. nonpregnant 1.56 vs. 0.95 vs. 0.85 and 0.746 μg/dL [36]
	(n = 470)	Canadian general population/Maternal blood AM Mn during pregnancy at delivery vs. nonpregnant; 2.4 vs. (0.8–1.2) μg/dL [37]
	(n = 1085)	USA general population/blood GM Mn in pregnancy vs. nonpregnant; 1.19 vs. 1.02 μg/dL [32]
	(n = 265)	Korean general population/blood GM Mn in pregnancy; 2.25 μg/dL [38]

AM, arithmetic mean; GM, geometric mean; KNHANES, Korea National Health and Nutrition Examination Survey; NHANES, National Health and Nutrition Examination Survey [22].
*Statistically significant.

Table 1. Behavior of blood manganese (Mn) concentrations according to gender-related variables.

Many cross-sectional studies have found that iron-deficiency anemia in children is associated with poor cognitive development, poor motor development, and behavioral problems due to the increased uptake of lead [23, 24]. There is also evidence that decreased cognitive development of children with iron deficiency persists after iron treatment and correction of anemia [23, 24]. Approximately 90% of the lead in the body is stored in the skeleton [40], and lead in bones has a half-life ranging from years (trabecular bone) to decades (cortical bone).

Several previous studies have assessed the temporal relationship between iron deficiency and increased blood lead concentration [15, 16, 41]. A longitudinal study showed an association between iron deficiency and high blood lead level in young children who had blood lead levels ranging from less than 5 to 40 μg/dL [42]. Another study of children aged 10–15 years reported the mean blood lead concentration was 6.9 μg/dL in iron-deficient children and 4.3 μg/dL in those with normal iron levels, and that iron supplementation significantly decreased blood lead concentrations in the former group [16]. A clinical trial assessing the impact of iron supplementation on blood lead concentrations in infants with iron deficiency found that blood lead concentration decreased as iron status improved [15, 41]. In contrast to these studies, other studies have found no association between iron deficiency and increased blood lead concentration [42–46].

This discrepancy may be partly due to the different ages of the study subjects and the extent of their exposures to lead. For example, studies of older female children or adolescents reported no association of blood iron and lead levels [42, 44, 47]. Postmenarcheal women have lower blood lead concentrations than men, because estrogen promotes bone mineralization and redistributes blood lead into bone, and this estrogen effect overshadows the increasing effect of ferritin on blood lead level [48]. Hence, there is no association between high blood lead level and iron deficiency in postmenarcheal adolescents [48]. Some studies of children with lower blood lead concentrations (11.0 and 11.4 μg/dL) reported no association of blood lead and iron levels [43, 45]. However, longitudinal studies of children with blood lead levels in a similar age range reported an association between iron status and blood lead concentration following iron supplementation [16, 41]. Furthermore, we recently showed that blood lead levels are elevated among iron-deficient infants with very low blood lead concentrations (1.416–1.846 μg/dL) [15]; moreover, iron therapy significantly decreased the blood lead levels of iron deficient infants [12]. Even minor increases in blood lead concentration due to iron deficiency may have clinical implications in children, considering the lack of evidence that any level of lead in the blood can be considered safe [26].

2.3. Cadmium

Cadmium is a ubiquitous environmental pollutant, and the main environmental sources are air, soil, and water contamination due to industrial activities, use of phosphate fertilizers, combustion of motor fuels, and particles released by tire wear. Smoking is the most important source, because tobacco plants, like other plants, take up cadmium from soil. In nonsmokers, diet is the major source of cadmium exposure [49]. Cadmium increases the risk of overall mortality and cardiovascular including hypertension, neurologic, renal, and developmental diseases in adults [49]. A recent paper showed that prenatal low-level exposure to cadmium had adverse effects on neurodevelopment in children [50]. Cadmium levels in the body increase with age, because only small amounts (0.01–0.02%) are excreted each day [49]. Blood cadmium is a biomarker of recent exposure, and urinary cadmium is a biomarker of lifetime exposure [49].

The body absorbs iron and cadmium by similar mechanisms [6, 22], and animal experiments have shown there may be metabolic interactions between cadmium and iron [6, 22]. In particular, animals with low iron stores have increased cadmium uptake [18, 20, 51]. Moreover, high cadmium concentrations are present in premenopausal women with low iron stores [33, 42, 52–55]. Females of childbearing age have higher blood cadmium concentrations than males because of their lower ferritin levels [53, 56–61]. There is also a significant increase in the whole blood cadmium level during late pregnancy in particular [53, 62–64] (**Table 2**). This increase may be caused by an enhanced cadmium absorption due to upregulated iron absorption during late pregnancy [53], because the mechanisms of iron absorption are similar to those of other divalent metals, particularly manganese and cadmium [6, 7]. However, there is no association between iron deficiency and elevated cadmium levels in postmenopausal women [60, 65, 66]. This may be because of the higher cadmium absorption rate in older-aged females than males, and the interaction of iron and cadmium uptake. Our recent study showed no association between iron deficiency and cadmium concentration in infants [67], but assessment of the same study subjects showed that iron deficiency was associated with increased blood lead and manganese concentrations [15, 30]. It is possible that the lower likelihood of exposure to cadmium in infants explains the lack of an association of blood cadmium level with iron deficiency in these individuals. The placenta may partially prevent

Variables	No. (n)	Study subjects and findings
Gender	(n = 7920)	US general population NHANES 2011–2012/ GM blood cadmium in men vs. women: 0.255 vs. 0.304 μg/L* [57]
	(n = 5924)	Korean general population aged 20 years or more; KNHANES 2008–2010/GM blood cadmium in men vs. women: 0.780 vs. 1.194 μg/L* [56]
	(n = 2257)	US general population aged 6 years and older; NHANES 2003–2004 / GM urinary cadmium in men aged 12 years or older lower than women; but no difference in children aged 6–11 [58]
	(n = 1055)	Bangladesh general population aged 8 years and older/Median urinary cadmium in men aged 30–50, 51–88 years vs. women; 0.66 vs. 0.81, 0.88 vs. 1.1 μg/L [59]
Menopause	(n = 3700)	Korean general population/ blood GM cadmium in premenopause vs. postmenopause: 0.995 vs. 1.165 μg/L* [60]
	(n = 149)	Bangladesh general population aged more than 51 years/median urinary cadmium in women vs. men; 1.1 vs. 0.88 μg/L [59]
	(n = 1670)	German general population aged 25 or older/between-gender differences in blood GM cadmium greater in subjects >50 than <50 years of age [61]
Pregnancy	(n = 120)	Spain general population/No significant changes in urinary GM cadmium during pregnancy and postpartum; 0.44 vs. 0.64 μg/L [62]
	(n = 2882)	Chinese general population/Significant changes in the blood median cadmium between during late pregnancy and nonpregnancy; 0.75 vs. 0.5 μg/L [63]
	(n = 281)	Bangladesh general population/Median blood cadmium increased 15% from early pregnancy (0.5 μg/L) to 6 months postpartum [64]
	(n = 216)	Swedish general population/Median blood cadmium increased 13% from early pregnancy (0.16 μg/L) to 3 months postpartum [53]

GM, geometric mean; KNHANES, Korea National Health and Nutrition Examination Survey; NHANES, National Health and Nutrition Examination Survey [22].

*Statistically significant.

Table 2. Behavior of blood/urine cadmium concentrations according gender-related variables.

fetal exposure to cadmium [68] and only 5–10% of maternal blood cadmium is transferred to human milk, because metallothionein binds to cadmium in blood cells [69]. Moreover, blood cadmium concentrations tend to increase with age [49, 70–72].

3. Toxicological implications

The effect of iron deficiency on blood concentrations of other divalent metals has several clinical and toxicological implications. First, the present paper emphasizes the importance of assessing the iron level and hematologic status of individuals for studies of environmental exposure to divalent metals (manganese, lead, and cadmium) in general populations. In particular, given the high prevalence of iron deficiency in children, iron deficiency status must be considered as an important factor affecting their susceptibility to heavy metal toxicity, especially for environmental health risk assessments of low exposure to these toxic metals. Second, our results also emphasize that exposure to neurotoxic metals may aggravate iron-related developmental and behavioral problems in children and lead to subclinical neuropsychological problems in adults.

4. Conclusions

The apical divalent metal transporter 1 (DMT1) and the iron exporter ferroportin 1 (FPN1) are responsible for the absorption of iron and other divalent metals (manganese, lead, and cadmium). Thus, an iron-deficient diet can lead to excess absorption of manganese, lead, and cadmium, and high blood concentrations of these metals. Relative to males and postmenopausal women, females of childbearing age have higher blood concentrations of manganese because of their lower blood concentrations of ferritin. Several previous studies reported a temporal relationship between iron deficiency and increased blood lead concentrations in children. Blood cadmium concentrations are higher in females of childbearing age because of their lower ferritin concentrations than in men.

Conflict of interest

The author declares no conflicts of interest.

Author details

Yangho Kim

Address all correspondence to: yanghokm@ulsan.ac.kr

Departments of Occupational and Environmental Medicine, Ulsan University Hospital, University of Ulsan College of Medicine, Ulsan, South Korea

References

[1] de Benoist B, McLean E, Egli I, Cogswell M. Worldwide Prevalence of Anaemia 1993-2005: WHO Global Database of Anaemia. Technical Report. Geneva: World Health Organization; 2008

[2] Centers for Disease Control and Prevention. Recommendations to prevent and control iron deficiency in the United States. Centers for Disease Control and Prevention. MMWR - Recommendations and Reports. 1998;**47**(RR-3):1-29

[3] World Health Organization. Iron Deficency Anaemia: Assessment, Prevention and Control: A Guide for Programme Managers. Geneva: World Health Organization; 2001

[4] Lucchini RG, Kim Y. Health effects of manganese. In: Vojtisek M, Prakash R, et al., editors. Metals and Neurotoxicity. India: Society for Science and Environment; 2009. pp. 119-147

[5] Lonnerdal B. Manganese nutrition of infants. In: Klimis-Tavantzis DJ, editor. Manganese in Health and Disease. Boca Raton: CRC Press; 1994. pp. 175-191

[6] Hurley LS, Keen CL. Manganese. In: Underwood E, Mertz W, editors. Trace Elements in Human Health and Animal Nutrition. New York: Academic Press; 1987. pp. 185-223

[7] Mackenzie B, Garrick MD. Iron imports. II. Iron uptake at the apical membrane in the intestine. American Journal of Physiology. Gastrointestinal and Liver Physiology. 2005;**289**:G981-G986

[8] Donovan A, Lima CA, Pinkus JL, Pinkus GS, Zon LI, Robine S, Andrews NC. The iron exporter ferroportin/Sc40a1 is essential for iron homeostasis. Cell Metabolism. 2005;**1**: 191-200

[9] Madejczyk MS, Ballatori N. The iron transporter ferroportin can also function as a manganese exporter. Biochimica et Biophysica Acta. 2012;**1818**:651-657

[10] Canonne-Hergaux F, Gruenheid S, Ponka P, Gros P. Cellular and subcellular localization of the Nramp2 iron transporter in the intestinal brush border and regulation by dietary iron. Blood. 1999;**93**:4406-4417

[11] Zoller H, Koch RO, Theurl I, et al. Expression of the duodenal iron transporters divalent-metal transporter 1 and ferroportin 1 in iron deficiency and iron overload. Gastroenterology. 2001;**120**:1412-1419

[12] Davis CD, Wolf TL, Greger JL. Varying levels of manganese and iron affect absorption and gut endogenous losses of manganese by rats. The Journal of Nutrition. 1992;**122**: 1300-1308

[13] Kim Y, Park JK, Choi Y, Yoo CI, Lee CR, Lee H, et al. Blood manganese concentration is elevated in iron deficiency anemia patients, whereas globus pallidus signal intensity is minimally affected. Neurotoxicology. 2005;**26**:107-111

[14] Kim Y, Lee BK. Iron deficiency increases blood manganese level in the Korean general population according to KNHANES 2008. Neurotoxicology. 2011;**32**:247-254

[15] Park S, Sim CS, Lee H, Kim Y. Effects of iron therapy on blood lead concentrations in infants. Journal of Trace Elements in Medicine and Biology. 2014;**28**:56-59

[16] Choi JW, Kim SK. Association between blood lead concentrations and body iron status in children. Archives of Disease in Childhood. 2003;**88**:791-792

[17] Watson WS, Hume R, Moore MR. Iron and lead absorption in humans. The American Journal of Clinical Nutrition. 1982;**36**:823-829

[18] Piasek M, Blanusa M, Kostial K, Laskey JW. Low iron diet and parenteral cadmium exposure in pregnant rats: The effects on trace elements and fetal viability. Biometals. 2004;**17**:1-14

[19] Tallkvist J, Bowlus CL, Lonnerdal B. DMT1 gene expression and cadmium absorption in human absorptive enterocytes. Toxicology Letters. 2001;**122**:171-177

[20] Ryu DY, Lee SJ, Park DW, Choi BS, Klaassen CD, Park JD. Dietary iron regulates intestinal cadmium absorption through iron transporters in rats. Toxicology Letters. 2004;**152**: 19-25

[21] Garrick MD, Dolan KG. An expression system for a transporter of iron and other metals. Methods in Molecular Biology. 2002;**196**:147-154

[22] Lee B-K, Kim Y. Sex-specific profiles of blood metal levels associated with metal–iron interactions. Safety and Health at Work. 2014;**5**:113-117

[23] Kim Y, Park S. Iron deficiency increases blood concentrations of neurotoxic metals in children. Korean Journal of Pediatrics. 2014;**57**:345-350

[24] Jeong KS, Park H, Ha E, Hong YC, Ha M, Park H, Kim BN, Lee SJ, Lee KY, Kim JH, Kim Y. Evidence that cognitive deficit in children is associated not only with iron deficiency, but also with blood lead concentration: A preliminary study. Journal of Trace Elements in Medicine and Biology. 2015;**29**:336-341

[25] ATSDR. Toxicological Profile for Manganese. Atlanta, GA: Agency for Toxic Substances and Disease Registry; 2012

[26] Bellinger DC. Prenatal exposures to environmental chemicals and children's neurodevelopment: An update. Safety and Health at Work. 2013;**4**:1-11

[27] Erikson KM, Shihabi ZK, Aschner JL, Aschner M. Manganese accumulates in iron-deficient rat brain regions in a heterogeneous fashion and is associated with neurochemical alterations. Biological Trace Element Research. 2002;**87**:143-156

[28] Boojar MM, Goodarzi F, Basedaghat MA. Long-term follow-up of workplace and well water manganese effects on iron status indexes in manganese miners. Archives of Environmental Health. 2002;**57**:519-528

[29] Brna P, Gordon K, Dooley JM, Price V. Manganese toxicity in a child with iron deficiency and polycythemia. Journal of Child Neurology. 2011;**26**:891-894

[30] Park S, Sim CS, Lee H, Kim Y. Blood manganese concentration is elevated in infants with iron deficiency. Biological Trace Element Research. 2013;**155**:184-189

[31] Baldwin M, Mergler D, Larribe F, Bélanger S, Tardif R, Bilodeau L, Hudnell K. Bioindicator and exposure data for a population based study of manganese. Neurotoxicology. 1999; **20**:343-353

[32] Oulhote Y, Mergler D, Bouchard MF. Sex- and age-differences in blood manganese levels in the U.S. general population: National Health and Nutrition Examination Survey 2011-2012. Environmental Health. 2014;**13**:87

[33] Lee BK, Kim Y. Effects of menopause on blood manganese levels in women: Analysis of 2008-2009 Korean National Health and Nutrition Examination Survey Data. Neurotoxicology. 2012;**33**:401-405

[34] Tholin K, Sandström B, Palm R, Hallmans G. Changes in blood manganese levels during pregnancy in iron supplemented and non supplemented women. Journal of Trace Elements in Medicine and Biology. 1995;**9**:13-17

[35] Spencer A. Whole blood manganese levels in pregnancy and the neonate. Nutrition. 1999;**15**:731-734

[36] Takser L, Lafond J, Bouchard M, St-Amour G, Mergler D. Manganese levels during pregnancy and at birth: Relation to environmental factors and smoking in a Southwest Quebec population. Environmental Research. 2004;**95**:119-125

[37] Zota AR, Ettinger AS, Bouchard M, Amarasiriwardena CJ, Schwartz J, Hu H, Wright RO. Maternal blood manganese levels and infant birth weight. Epidemiology. 2009;**20**: 367-373

[38] Chung SE, Cheong H-K, Ha E-H, Kim B-N, Ha M, Kim Y, Hong Y-C, Park H, Oh S-Y. Maternal blood manganese and early neurodevelopment: The Mothers and Children's Environmental Health (MOCEH) Study. Environmental Health Perspectives. 2015;**123**: 717-722

[39] Kirchgessner M, Sherif YS, Schwarz FJ. Changes in absorption of manganese during gravidity and lactation. Annals of Nutrition & Metabolism. 1982;**26**:83-89. [in German]

[40] ATSDR. Toxicological profile for lead. Atlanta, GA: Agency for Toxic Substances and Disease Registry; 2007

[41] Wright RO, Tsaih SW, Schwartz J, Wright RJ, Hu H. Association between iron deficiency and blood lead level in a longitudinal analysis of children followed in an urban primary care clinic. The Journal of Pediatrics. 2003;**142**:9-14

[42] Barany E, Bergdahl IA, Bratteby LE, Lundh T, Samuelson G, Skerfving S, et al. Iron status influences trace element levels in human blood and serum. Environmental Research. 2005;**98**:215-223

[43] Hammad TA, Sexton M, Langenberg P. Relationship between blood lead and dietary iron intake in preschool children. A cross-sectional study. Annals of Epidemiology. 1996;**6**:30-33

[44] Hershko C, Konijn AM, Moreb J, Link G, Grauer F, Weissenberg E. Iron depletion and blood lead levels in a population with endemic lead poisoning. Israel Journal of Medical Sciences. 1984;**20**:1039-1043

[45] Wolf AW, Jimenez E, Lozoff B. No evidence of developmental III effects of low-level lead exposure in a developing country. Journal of Developmental and Behavioral Pediatrics. 1994;**15**:224-231

[46] Clark M, Royal J, Seeler R. Interaction of iron deficiency and lead and the hematologic findings in children with severe lead poisoning. Pediatrics. 1988;**81**:247-254

[47] Yip R, Dallman PR. Developmental changes in erythrocyte protoporphyrin: Roles of iron deficiency and lead toxicity. The Journal of Pediatrics. 1984;**104**:710-713

[48] Sim CS, Kim Y, Lee H, Park CY, Ham JO, Lee BK. Iron deficiency increases blood lead levels in boys and pre-menarche girls surveyed in KNHANES 2010-2011. Environmental Research. 2014;**130**:1-6

[49] ATSDR. Toxicological Profile for Cadmium. Atlanta, GA: Agency for Toxic Substances and Disease Registry; 2008

[50] Jeong KS, Park H, Ha E, Hong YC, Ha M, Park H, Kim BN, Lee BE, Lee SJ, Lee KY, Kim JH, Kim Y. Performance IQ in children is associated with blood cadmium concentration in early pregnancy. Journal of Trace Elements in Medicine and Biology. 2015;**30**:107-111

[51] Flanagan PR, McLellan JS, Haist J, Cherian G, Chamberlain MJ, Valberg LS. Increased dietary cadmium absorption in mice and human subjects with iron deficiency. Gastroenterology. 1978;**74**:841-846

[52] Vahter M, Berglund M, Akesson A, Liden C. Metals and women's health. Environmental Research. 2002;**88**:145-155

[53] Åkesson A, Berglund M, Schütz A, Bjellerup P, Bremme K, Vahter M. Cadmium exposure in pregnancy and lactation in relation to iron status. American Journal of Public Health. 2002;**92**:284-287

[54] Berglund M, Akesson A, Nermell B, Vahter M. Intestinal absorption of dietary cadmium in women depends on body iron stores and fiber intake. Environmental Health Perspectives. 1994;**102**:1058-1066

[55] Gallagher CM, Chen JJ, Kovach JS. The relationship between body iron stores and blood and urine cadmium concentrations in US never-smoking, non-pregnant women aged 20-49 years. Environmental Research. 2011;**111**:702-707

[56] Kim Y, Lee BK. Associations of blood lead, cadmium, and mercury with estimated glomerular filtration rate in the Korean general population: Analysis of 2008-2010 Korean

National Health and Nutrition Examination Survey Data. Environmental Research. 2012;**118**:124-129

[57] Centers for Disease Control and Prevention. Fourth National Report on Human Exposure to Environmental Chemicals; 2018. p. 285 [Accessed: May 12, 2018]

[58] Ruiz P, Mumtaz M, Osterloh J, Fisher J, Fowler BA. Interpreting NHANES biomonitoring data, cadmium. Toxicology Letters. 2010;**198**:44-48

[59] Berglund M, Lindberg AL, Rahman M, Yunus M, Grandér M, Lönnerdal B, Vahter M. Gender and age differences in mixed metal exposure and urinary excretion. Environmental Research. 2011;**111**:1271-1279

[60] Kim SH, Kim Y, Kim NS, Lee BK. Gender difference in blood cadmium concentration in the general population: Can it be explained by iron deficiency? Journal of Trace Elements in Medicine and Biology. 2014;**28**:322-327

[61] Hoffmann K, Krause C, Seifert B. The German Environmental Survey 1990/92 (GerES II): Primary predictors of blood cadmium levels in adults. Archives of Environmental Health. 2001;**56**:374-379

[62] Hernandez M, Schuhmacher M, Fernandez JD, Domingo JL, Llobet JM. Urinary cadmium levels during pregnancy and postpartum. A longitudinal study. Biological Trace Element Research. 1996;**53**:205-212

[63] Zhang Z, Yuan E, Liu J, Lou X, Jia L, Li X, Zhang L. Gestational age-specific reference intervals for blood copper, zinc, calcium, magnesium, iron, lead, and cadmium during normal pregnancy. Clinical Biochemistry. 2013;**46**:777-780

[64] Kippler M, Goessler W, Nermell B, Ekström EC, Lönnerdal B, El Arifeen S, Vahter M. Factors influencing intestinal cadmium uptake in pregnant Bangladeshi women—A prospective cohort study. Environmental Research. 2009;**109**:914-921

[65] Horiguchi H, Oguma E, Sasaki S, Miyamoto K, Ikeda Y, Machida M, et al. Comprehensive study of the effects of age, iron deficiency, diabetes mellitus, and cadmium burden on dietary cadmium absorption in cadmium-exposed female Japanese farmers. Toxicology and Applied Pharmacology. 2004;**196**:114-123

[66] Tsukahara T, Ezaki T, Moriguchi J, Furuki K, Fukui Y, Ukai H, et al. No significant effect of iron deficiency on cadmium body burden or kidney dysfunction among women in the general population in Japan. International Archives of Occupational and Environmental Health. 2003;**76**:275-281

[67] Park JH, Park S, Kim Y. Iron deficiency is not associated with increased blood cadmium in infants. Annals of Occupational and Environmental Medicine. 2014;**26**:3

[68] Truska P, Rosival L, Balazova G, Hinst J, Rippel A, Palusova O, et al. Blood and placental concentrations of cadmium, lead, and mercury in mothers and their newborns. Journal of Hygiene, Epidemiology, Microbiology, and Immunology. 1989;**33**:141-147

[69] Radisch B, Luck W, Nau H. Cadmium concentrations in milk and blood of smoking mothers. Toxicology Letters. 1987;**36**:147-152

[70] Olsson IM, Bensryd I, Lundh T, Ottosson H, Skerfving S, Oskarsson A. Cadmium in blood and urine: Impact of sex, age, dietary intake, iron status, and former smoking: Association of renal effects. Environmental Health Perspectives. 2002;**110**:1185-1190

[71] Lee BK, Kim Y. Iron deficiency is associated with increased levels of blood cadmium in the Korean general population: Analysis of 2008-2009 Korean National Health and Nutrition Examination Survey Data. Environmental Research. 2012;**112**:155-163

[72] Centers for Disease Control and Prevention. NHANES, Key Statistics From NHANES (Data are for 2003-2006) [Internet]. Atlanta, GA: US Centers for Disease Control and Prevention. [Cited 2012 Dec 1]. Available from: http://wwwn.cdc.gov/nchs/nhanes/bibliography/key_statistics.asp

Chapter 4

Vegetal Sources of Iron

Elia Hermila Valdes-Miramontes,
Ramon Rodriguez-Macias and Mario Ruiz-Lopez

Additional information is available at the end of the chapter

http://dx.doi.org/10.5772/intechopen.79834

Abstract

Iron deficiency anemia is a global public health problem. According to the World Health Organization, anemia affects 1620 million of people worldwide, which corresponds to 28% of the population. Fifty percent of the anemia cases are attributed to low iron intake. Among the main sources of iron from vegetable origin are legumes, such as beans, lentils, soybeans, lupin, some vegetables such as spinach, and some dehydrated fruits. Non-hemic iron is mainly from legumes and is the most important source of this mineral in the diet of developing countries' population, but its bioavailability is very variable. Consequently, the fortification of foods with high and cheap iron sources is a practical way to prevent its deficiency. Some studies have shown that the roots of some legumes, especially nitrogen fixers, accumulate a significant amount of iron mainly in the nodule proteins. The purpose of this chapter is to present the current knowledge of novel sources of plant-based hemic iron with a high bioavailability to be used in food fortification.

Keywords: plants, iron, anemia, fortification

1. Introduction

Iron deficiency affects an important part of the human population; it is the most common nutritional disorder and causes approximately 50% of anemia cases. The groups most likely to have iron deficiency and iron deficiency anemia are infants, young children, adolescents, premenopausal women, and especially pregnant women. The recommended iron intake depends on the individual's health status, age, and sex. However, some sociodemographic factors such as race or ethnicity, socioeconomic status, eating habits, etc. have an influence on the risk of developing anemia. Iron deficiency and iron deficiency anemia have undesirable physiological consequences especially in children, having an impact on cognitive performance and growth [1].

IntechOpen

© 2018 The Author(s). Licensee IntechOpen. This chapter is distributed under the terms of the Creative Commons Attribution License (http://creativecommons.org/licenses/by/3.0), which permits unrestricted use, distribution, and reproduction in any medium, provided the original work is properly cited.

This pathology decreases the amount of oxygen transported to the muscles, which affects people's physical capacity and work performance. It generates a decrease in the immune system response and therefore an increased risk of contracting infections. Iron deficiency also disrupts the digestive system functioning. During pregnancy, iron deficiency anemia increases the perinatal risk of both mothers and children and can lead to an increase in infant mortality. From the biochemical point of view, it has been observed that it affects the metabolism of some neurotransmitters, thyroid hormones, and the activity of some iron-dependent enzymes. Due to the great impact of iron deficiency and iron deficiency anemia on human health and its high incidence, international organizations led by the World Health Organization have developed a series of programs to avoid this problem [2].

In developed countries, iron deficiency is usually a consequence of absorption disorders, loss of blood, or the intake of a restricted diet (vegan diet). Foods present different forms of iron that differ in their bioavailability, depending to the source. Hemic iron is present mainly in animal proteins such as hemoglobin and myoglobin, which has a higher bioavailability; these proteins are present in meat, fish, and shellfish [3].

Non-hemic iron is present in different chemical forms, which significantly affects its absorption. This type of iron is present in both organic and inorganic forms. The most common sources of non-hemic iron present in foods are low-molecular-weight compounds such as ferric citrate, phosphate, phytate, oxalate, and hydroxide and high-molecular-weight compounds such as ferritin, lactoferrin, and leghemoglobin. The best sources of non-hemic iron are seeds, grains, nuts, and the green leaves of vegetables [3, 4].

Likewise, the absorption of iron depends to a large extent on the concentration of iron present in the body and enhancers such as ascorbic acid and some muscle tissue proteins. One of the strategies for the replenishment of iron deficiency is the use of food supplements. However, the World Health Organization recommends fortification of foods as an approach to increase iron intake [5].

2. Iron biological functions

Iron is an essential metal for human life, and its main biological function is as a part of the heme group proteins such as hemoglobin and myoglobin, which is responsible for oxygen transport [6]; also, iron is an essential component of many enzymes that catalyze redox reactions, due to its ability to rapidly accept electrons, under physiological conditions [7].

More than 2 billion people worldwide suffer from anemia. Iron deficiency anemia is the most common nutritional disease in the world; around 800 million children and women are the most vulnerable and suffer from this type of anemia, which can affect the physical and immune development [3, 8]. This disease is usually asymptomatic and is often not diagnosed; however, some of its symptoms are weakness, fatigue, exhaustion, and decreased cognitive efficiency [9]. The iron status in the body is maintained by a complex process that regulates the balance between iron absorption in the duodenum, the recycling of iron by macrophages and iron storage in the liver because there is no physiological way for its excretion [10]. Hemic

http://dx.doi.org/10.5772/intechopen.79834

iron is present in foods of animal origin and in some plants proteins, such as leghemoglobin present in legume nodules; however, non-hemic iron is mainly present in foods such as vegetables [6].

3. Iron absorption

The absorption of iron is defined as the passage from the intestinal lumen to the circulation through the enterocytes and is mainly carried out in the duodenum and the proximal jejunum [11]. Non-hemic iron must be in a soluble form to be absorbed, since the insoluble forms cannot be absorbed and are eliminated with the feces. The ferrous forms of iron are much more soluble than ferric forms, since the latter rapidly precipitate in the intestine alkaline medium. That is why iron that has been released by the action of gastric and pancreatic proteases binds to intraluminal ligands whose function is to stabilize the ferrous form, keeping the iron soluble and consequently biologically available to be captured and transferred to the interior of the enterocyte [12].

The non-hemic iron complexes present in foods are degraded during digestion in the gastrointestinal tract due to the action of pepsin and hydrochloric acid. Once released from the food components, most non-hemic iron is present in the ferric form (Fe^{+3}) which is more common in vegetables, it is considered to be of low solubility and bioavailability, but this depends on the physiological status and the presence of other minerals such as zinc, magnesium, copper, and calcium [13], as well as phytates, polyphenols, and metal chelators. In addition, there are numerous compounds present in foods capable of reducing Fe^{+3} and Fe^{+2} (bioavailable non-hemic iron form), including ascorbic acid and amino acids such as cysteine and histidine, and

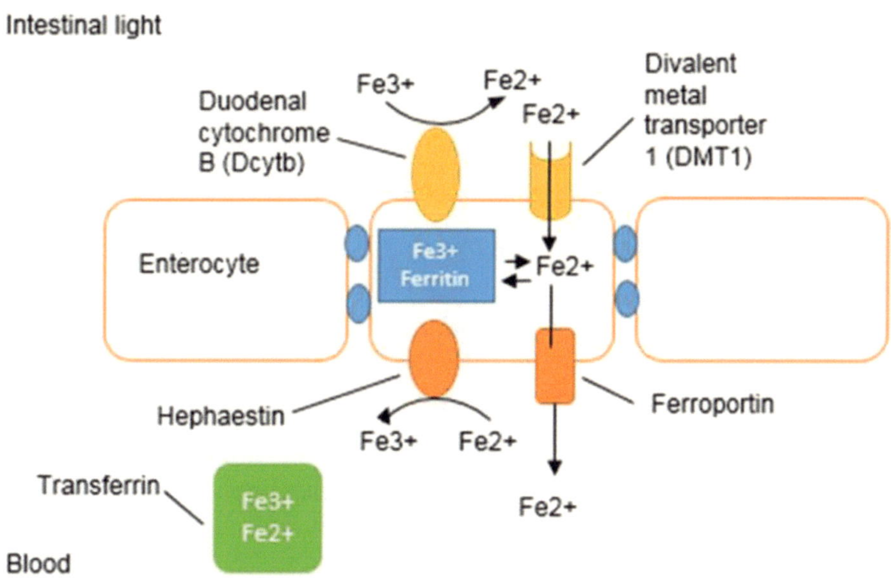

Figure 1. Iron uptake in the apical enterocyte membrane [8].

also, the main reduction activity is carried out by duodenal cytochrome b reductase activity (DCYTB), a hemoprotein located in the enterocyte apical membrane using ascorbate to facilitate iron reduction [14]. The soluble form of Fe^{+2} is transported to the enterocyte through the divalent metal transporter-1 (DMT-1), which is a proton simulator that requires a low pH for metal transport (**Figure 1**) [15].

4. Vegetable sources of iron and its bioavailability

Non-hemic iron includes different organic forms, such as ferric citrate, ferric gluconate, ferrous fumarate, and ferritin and inorganic forms such as ferrous sulfate, carbonate, and chloride as well as ferric, and each form of iron has different forms of absorption and efficiencies [16] and is mainly found in legumes, cereals, and other vegetables (**Table 1**).

Legumes throughout the history have been a very important food resource, accounting for approximately 20% of the daily protein intake in humans. They are also an economical source of dietary fiber and minerals such as iron [17, 18].

The iron in food is found as hemic iron, forming part of the structure of proteins and as non-hemic iron. The most common forms of non-hemic iron present in foods are low-molecular-weight compounds such as ferric citrate, phosphate, phytate, oxalate, and hydroxide [19].

Hemic iron is also present in vegetables forming part of some proteins such as ferritin and leghemoglobin. The distribution of ferritin in the edible parts of plants is variable. Its concentration in seeds can range from 50 to 70 mg/kg, which corresponds to the iron content of 10 mg/kg [20].

Both ferritin and leghemoglobin accumulate in the nodules of the root of legumes such as soybean and lupine. The concentration of iron in the nodules of soy is high compared to the leaves [21].

Valdés-Miramontes et al. [22] reported a concentration of iron in the seed of *L. rotundiflorus* of 6.12 mg/100 g and a concentration of 70 mg/100 g in the whole root; this concentration in nodules is probably due to the fact that the root has nodules rich in leghemoglobin, an iron-rich protein, due to its high activity in nitrogen fixation. Leghemoglobin hemoprotein is found in root nodules of legumes, containing high concentrations of iron [23].

Values obtained from the "Table of practical use of foods with the highest consumption" by Chávez et al. [24] and "Effect of thermal treatment on the chemical composition and minerals of wild lupine seeds" by Valdés-Miramontes et al. [20].

In a study conducted by Martínez-Zavala et al. [25] about the iron content in the bean plant leaves *(Phaseolus vulgaris)*, a recovery of hematic biomarkers was observed, such as hemoglobin, erythrocyte count, and hematocrit in rats with induced anemia, when diets with iron source from this legume were administered.

It is known as bioavailability of iron to the proportion of this dietary mineral that is absorbed and used by the body. **Figures 2** and **3** show some of the dietary and physiological factors that influence the bioavailability of iron in foods [6, 8].

Food	Iron (mg / 100 g)	Humidity (g / 100 g)
Pumpkin seed (*Cucurbita pepo*)	14	4.07
Soy (*Glycine max*)	13.70	
Sunflower seed (Helianthus annus L).	5.25	4.80
Cocoa (*Theobroma cacao L.*)	3. 4	3.60
Lentils (*Lens succulent*)	5.80	7.86
Bean (*Phaseolus) vulgaris L.*)	5.70	10.10
Bean flour	13.50	
Chickpea (*Cicer arietinum L.)*	8.90	8.10
Bean flour (*Vicia faba*)	18.20	4.70
Soybeans, cooked seed	15.70	
Green Creole pumpkin (*Cucurbita pepo*)	22	91
Cilantro (*Coriandrum) sativum L.*)	6.10	90.1
Endive leaf (*Cichorium endivia*)	12.5	94.5
Parsley (*Petroselinum sativum*)	6.20	80
Leeks (*Allium porum L.)*	28	82.7
Quelite or Chinese spinach (*Amaranthuschlorostachys*)	6.20	
Pepermint (*Mentha sativa L.*)	7.5	85
Chives (*Allimun porum*)	8.40	94
L. albus	8.06	7.5
L. angustifolius	7.6	7.9
L. mutabilis	1.08	8.0
L. exaltatus	6.18	7.4
L. elegans	7.09	7.1
L. mexicanus	6.31	7.5
L. montanus	7.77	7.2
L. rotundiflorus	8.28	7.8
Root of *L. rotundiflorus*	70.0	0.0

Table 1. Iron content (mg) and moisture in different foods.

Recent research on iron bioavailability from legume ferritin, especially soy ferritin, suggests a high bioavailability of soy ferritin, comparable to the bioavailability of $FeSO_4$, on in vitro experiments, rat assays, and clinical studies. This is probably due to the fact that the root presents nodules that contain leghemoglobin, a protein rich in hemic iron [3, 8].

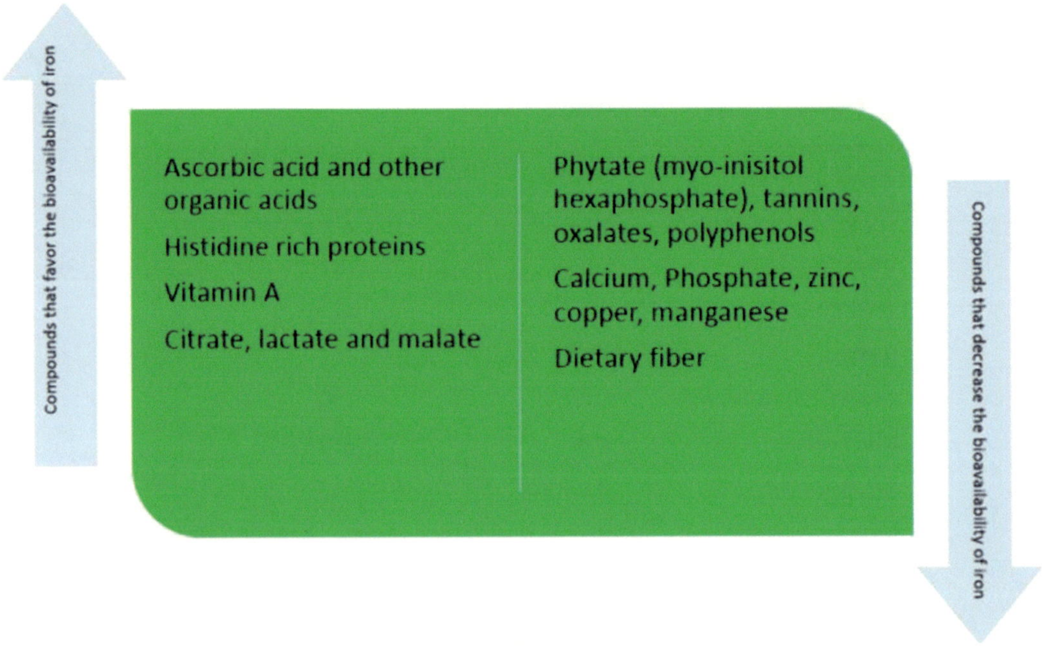

Figure 2. Dietary factors that influence the bioavailability of iron in foods.

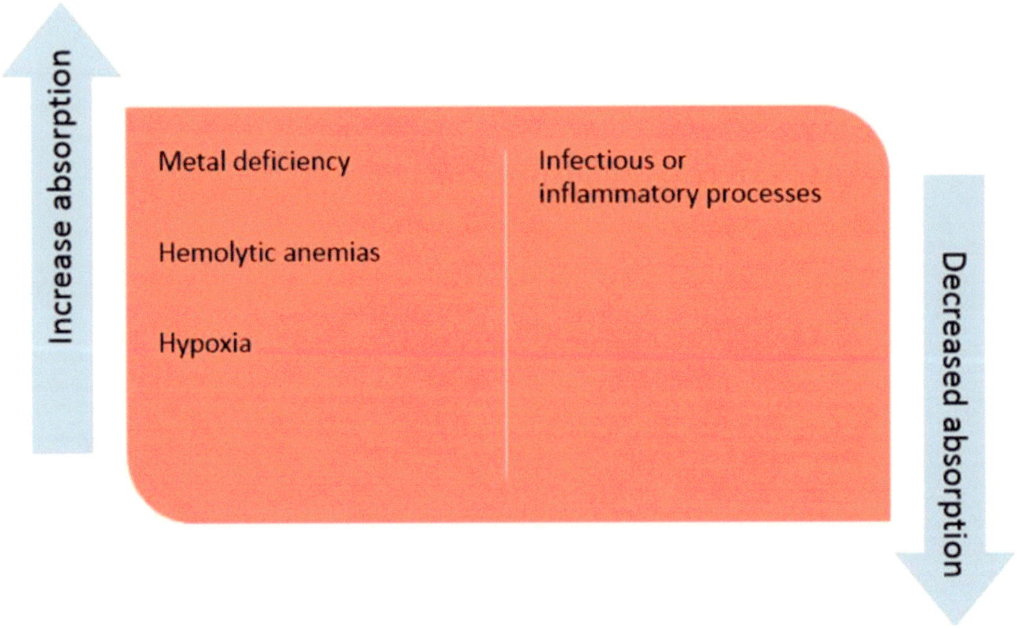

Figure 3. Physiological factors that influence the bioavailability of iron in foods [3, 8].

In this way, Proulx and Reddy [26] report an iron bioavailability from soybean nodules of 28 ± 10% and a partially purified soybean leghemoglobin bioavailability of 19 ± 17%, with a relative biological value (RBV) of 125 and 113, respectively, with a reference to ferrous sulfate (considered as 100%).When 50 ppm of partially purified leghemoglobin soybean extracts and bovine hemoglobin were added to corn tortillas, bioavailability was 27 and 33%, respectively [26].

It has been reported that iron bioavailability in bean leaves is 8.5%, while fava beans reported an absorption rate of 37.10 for a basal diet supplemented with 21 g of dry thyme leaves/kg of diet that contributed a concentration of iron 70.67 ppm [27, 28].

Valdés-Miramontes et al. [22] reported that the bioavailability of iron in the root nodules and cooked seeds of *L. rotundiflorus* of 13.80 and 13.70%, respectively, evaluated through the depletion hemoglobin repletion method in Wistar strain rats.

5. Fortification of foods with vegetable iron

Because of the importance of Fe deficiencies in health, the study of plants with higher content of bioavailable Fe is crucial, as biofortification which is considered as an innovative strategy for the micronutrient malnutrition in a sustainable way, since the micronutrients' deficiency is responsible for what is known as silent malnutrition, in particular iron deficiency, which has adverse effects on growth, immune function and causes anemia [29].

Figure 4 represents the three strategies to diminish iron deficiency in the population.

Biofortification is the process of improving micronutrient content of crops base to our feeding, through fertilization, breeding, and use of genetically modified varieties, comparing the cost-benefit and long-term sustainability, which can help increase the daily intake of micronutrients to low-income populations. Biofortification is a feasible means for malnourished populations in rural areas, offering naturally fortified foods to people with limited access to commercialized fortified foods, which are more available in urban areas. The biofortification and commercial fortification are highly complementary [30].

Biofortification is a novel strategy for producing crops with high micronutrient contents, and it reduces the levels of antinutritional factors that promote the increase of substances that promote nutrient absorption [31].

There is still ignorance regarding important parts of the biofortification process, also effectiveness more trials are needed to identify and refine the nutrients synergies. Additionally, more marketing strategies must be done to ensure maximum consumption of biofortified crops. Improvement can be made more cost-effective by selecting high levels of vitamins and minerals from a single variety, and transgenic methods can be more effective with conventional breeding crops [32].

In this way, Miller et al. [33] suggest to follow the next recommendations:

1. Commercially expand fortified food programs as a strategy to prevent micronutrient malnutrition (iron).
2. Develop and implement technologies to fortify foods, with the purpose of increasing the micronutrients consumption, especially in rural populations of developing countries.
3. Reduce the loss of food and food waste, especially in fruits and vegetables that should be used in a sustainable manner.
4. Training in agriculture, food processing, and nutrition education, especially in developing countries and their rural areas.

Velu et al. [34] report that a strategy of fertilization combined with genetic improvement in wheat enriches this crop with high iron content of high availability.

The improvement in popular consumption plants would be through increasing the concentration of absorption promoters such as nicotianamine, ascorbic acid, inulin, and carotenes.

Much research has been done recently regarding nicotianamine specifically, suggesting that genetic engineering is likely to have an even greater potential for biofortification, since nicotianamine concentrations in transgenic plants exceed the range found naturally, which would be complemented by studies concerning nicotianamine efficiency in human consumption.

Since it has been observed an enhancing effect of nicotianamine on the absorption of Fe by intestinal epithelial cells during passage through the human or digestive system, the continuation of research along these and other pathways will soon lead to even more effective and sustainable biofortification solutions [35].

Recently, new technologies have emerged with significant advances in iron biofortification programs. These include mutagenesis oligo-directed, reverse reproduction, DNA methylation directed by RNA, and specific sequence technology nuclease or genome edition. These

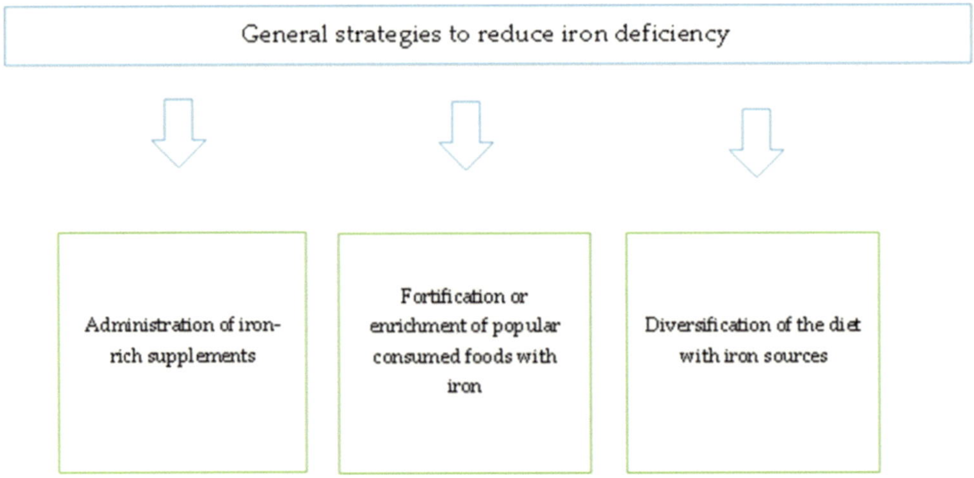

Figure 4. General strategies to reduce iron deficiency [3].

technologies have obtained very fast benefits and at low cost. At this time, it is a common practice to combine different molecular crops and genomic methods such as marker-assisted selection [36].

Recent success stories can be found in www.HarvestPlus.org.

Additionally, the use of ferritin is currently being explored as a strategy in iron supplementation or biofortification, which showed by Lv et al. [37] in a study of in vitro and in vivo digestibility (with Caco-2 cells).

6. Conclusions

Iron deficiency is a big health problem that affects a large proportion of the world's population, especially in developing countries, causing what is known as "hidden malnutrition." In this chapter, the importance of iron is mentioned, as well as its functions within the organism as an oxygen transporter and forming part of some enzymes. The absorption of this mineral depends on several factors such as the ferrous forms, hemic and non-hemic, presence of other minerals, phytates, and some polyphenols. Plant-based foods commonly contain non-hemic Fe, which is considered to be of low solubility and bioavailability; however, some plants contain hemic Fe, forming part of proteins such as ferritin and leghemoglobin, also some plant foods contain high amounts of Fe as pumpkins, cocoa, and various legumes such as beans, soybeans, fava beans, especially their roots that form nodules with bacteria, which will convert atmospheric nitrogen to form soluble by the plant; consequently, they have a large amount of leghemoglobin, which is an oxygen carrier protein and rich in hemic Fe.

Likewise, strategies to reduce iron deficiency are mentioned, as well as the diversification of foods rich in this mineral, supplementation, and fortification of popular consumed foods enriched in Fe. One of the strategies that has worked so far is the biofortification of staple crops in rural areas in developing countries, with high iron contents and low levels of absorption inhibitor compounds. The biofortification is done through the combination of fertilization with conventional genetic or transgenic improvement that enriches crops with high iron content of high bioavailability, which is estimated that more than 20 million people in developing countries consume biofortified crops.

Acknowledgements

This research was supported by the University of Guadalajara. The authors also thank the Doctoral Program in BEMARENA Biosystematic, Ecology and Management of Natural Resources, University of Guadalajara.

Conflict of interest

The authors declare no conflict of interest.

Author contributions

All authors participated in the analysis of information and write and corrections of this chapter.

Author details

Elia Hermila Valdes-Miramontes[1], Ramon Rodriguez-Macias[2] and Mario Ruiz-Lopez[2*]

*Address all correspondence to: mruiz@cucba.udg.mx

1 CUSur, Behavioral Feeding and Nutrition Research Center (CICAN), University of Guadalajara, Ciudad Guzmán, Jalisco, México

2 Botanical and Zoology Department, University of Guadalajara, CUCBA, Biotechnology Laboratory, Zapopan, Jalisco, Mexico

References

[1] Abu-Ouf NM, Jan MM. The impact of maternal iron deficiency and iron deficiency anemia on child's health. Saudi Medical Journal. 2015;**36**(2):146-149. DOI: 10.15537/smj.2015.2.10289

[2] Hassan TH, Badr MA, Karam NA, et al. Impact of iron deficiency anemia on the function of the immune system in children. Medicine. 2016;**95**(47):e5395. DOI: 10.1097/MD.0000000000005395

[3] OMS. The Global Prevalence of Anaemia in 2011 [Internet]. Organización Mundial de la Salud; 2015. Available from: http://www.who.int/nutrition/publications/micronutrients/global_prevalence_anaemia_2011/en/

[4] Geissler C, Singh M. Iron, meat and health. Nutrients. 2011;**3**(3):283-316. DOI: 10.3390/nu3030283

[5] Abbaspour N, Hurrell R, Kelishadi R. Review on iron and its importance for human health. Journal of Research in Medical Sciences: The Official Journal of Isfahan University of Medical Sciences. 2014;**19**(2):164-174

[6] Blanco-Rojo R, Vaquero MP. Iron bioavailability from food fortification to precision nutrition. A review. Innovative Food Science and Emergency Technology [Internet]. 2018. Available from: http://linkinghub.elsevier.com/retrieve/pii/S1466856418300705

[7] Ganz T. Systemic iron homeostasis. Physiological Reviews. 2013;**93**(4):1721-1741. DOI: 10.1152/physrev.00008.2013

[8] Brigide P, AtaideTda R, Canniatti-Brazaca SG, Baptista AS, Abdalla AL, Filho VFN, et al. Iron bioavailability of common beans (*Phaseolus vulgaris L.*) intrinsically labeled with 59Fe. Journal of Trace Elements in Medicine and Biology 2014;**28**(3):260-265

[9] Camaschella C. Iron-deficiency anemia. The New England Journal of Medicine. 2015; **372**(19):1832-1843. DOI: 10.1056/NEJMra1401038

[10] Rybinska I, Cairo G. Mutual cross talk between iron homeostasis and erythropoiesis. Vitamins and Hormones [Internet]. 2017;**105**:143-160. Available from: http://linkinghub.elsevier.com/retrieve/pii/S0083672917300018 [Accessed: Jun 19, 2018]

[11] Han O. Molecular mechanism of intestinal iron absorption. Metallomics. 2011;**3**(2):103. DOI: 10.1039/c0mt00043d

[12] Gomollón F, Gisbert JP. Anemia and inflammatory bowel diseases. World Journal of Gastroenterology. 2009;**15**(37):4659-4665. DOI: 10.3748/wjg.15.4659

[13] Hallberg L. Bioavailability of dietary iron in man. Annual Review of Nutrition. 1981; **1**(1):123-147. DOI: 10.1146/annurev.nu.01.070181.001011

[14] Sharp P, Srai S-K. Molecular mechanisms involved in intestinal iron absorption. World Journal of Gastroenterology. 2007;**13**(35):4716-4724

[15] De Domenico I, McVey Ward D, Kaplan J. Regulation of iron acquisition and storage: Consequences for iron-linked disorders. Nature Reviews Molecular Cell Biology. 2008; **9**(1):72-81. DOI: 10.1038/nrm2295

[16] Theil EC, Briat JF. Plant Ferritin and Non-heme Iron Nutrition in Humans. International Food Policy Research Institute and International Center for Tropical Agriculture (CIAT); 2004. Available from: https://pdfs.semanticscholar.org/a6c1/aaa7c9bcd53c46d6843a79f-5e4cd8c4f2f1b.pdf

[17] Garcia Y, Gonzalez M, Menendez R, Gonzalez R, Bourg V. Effect of supplementation with dehydrated formulation of iron + iron ion in rats. Journal of Food and Nutrition. 2008;**18**:204-212

[18] Guillamón E, García-Lafuente A, Lozano M, D'Arrigo M, Rostagno MA, Villares A, et al. Edible mushrooms: Role in the prevention of cardiovascular diseases. Fitoterapia. 2010; **81**(7):715-723

[19] Zielińska-Dawidziak M. Plant ferritin—A source of iron to prevent its deficiency. Nutrients. 2015;**7**(2):1184-1201. DOI: 10.3390/nu7021184

[20] Valdés-Miramontes EH, López-Espinoza A, Rodríguez-Macías R, Salcedo-Pérez E, Ruiz-López MA. Effect of thermal treatment on the chemical composition and minerals of wild lupin seeds.Revista Chilena de Nutrición. 2015;**42**(2):186-190. DOI: 10.1590/1678-98652017000600014

[21] Chungopast S, Duangkhet M, Tajima S, Ma JF, Nomura M. Iron-induced nitric oxide leads to an increase in the expression of ferritin during the senescence of Lotus japonicus nodules. Journal of Plant Physiology. 2017;**208**:40-46. DOI: 10.1016/j.jplph.2016.11.004

[22] Valdés-Miramontes EH, López-Espinoza A, Martínez Moreno AG, Zamora Natera JF, Rodríguez Macias R, Ruiz-Lopez MA. Iron bioavailability of *Lupinusrotundiflorus* seeds and roots in low-iron-diet treated rats. Revista de Nutrição. 2017;**30**(6):827-834. DOI: 10.1590/1678-98652017000600014

[23] Neudorf SJ. Reaction of the hemochromogen test with the heme protein leghemoglobin obtained from soybean root nodules. Canadian Society of Forensic Science Journal. 2015;**48**(1):36-45. DOI: 10.1080/00085030.2014.987474

[24] Chávez M. Tablas de usoprácticodel valor nutritivo de los alimentos de mayor consumo en México. México: McGraw Hill; 2014

[25] Martínez-Zavala M, Mora-Avilés MA, Anaya-Loyola MA, Guzmán-Maldonado H, Aguilera-Barreyro A, Blanco-Labra A, et al. Common bean leaves as a source of dietary iron: Functional test in an iron-deficient rat model. Plant foods for human nutrition (Dordrecht, Netherlands). 2016;**71**(3):259-264. DOI: 10.1007/s11130-016-0554-5

[26] Proulx AK, Reddy MB. Iron bioavailability of hemoglobin from soy root nodules using a Caco-2 cell culture model. Journal of Agricultural and Food Chemistry. 2006;**54**(4):1518-1522. DOI: 10.1021/jf052268l

[27] Rosado JL, Díaz M, González K, Griffin I, Abrams SA, Preciado R. The addition of milk or yogurt to a plant-based diet increases zinc bioavailability but does not affect iron bioavailability in women. Journal of Nutrition. 2005;**135**(3):465-468. DOI: 10.1093/jn/135.3.465

[28] Yossef HEE-D. Effect of calcium and phosphorus on nonhaeme iron absorption and haematogenic characteristics in rats. Food and Nutrition Sciences. 2010;**1**(1):13-18

[29] Murgia I, Arosio P, Tarantino D, Soave C. Biofortification for combating 'hidden hunger' for iron. Trends in Plant Science. 2012;**17**(1):47-55. DOI: 10.1016/j.tplants.2011.10.003

[30] Bouis HE, Hotz C, McClafferty B, Meenakshi JV, Pfeiffer WH. Biofortification: A new tool to reduce micronutrient malnutrition. Food and Nutrition Bulletin. 2011;**32** (1 Suppl):S31-S40. DOI: 10.1177/15648265110321S105

[31] Bouis HE. Micronutrient fortification of plants through plant breeding: Can it improve nutrition in man at low cost? Proceedings of the Nutrition Society. 2003;**62**(2):403-411

[32] Saltzman A, Birol E, Bouis HE, Boy E, DeMoura FF, Islam Y, Pfeiffer WH. Biofortification: Progress toward a more nourishing future. Global Food Security. 2013;**2**:9-12. DOI: 10.1016/j.gfs.2012.12.003

[33] Miller BDD, Welch RM. Food system strategies for preventing micronutrient malnutrition. Food Policy. 2013;**42**:115-128. DOI: 10.1016/j.foodpol.2013.06.008

[34] Velu G, Ortiz-Monasterio I, Cakmak I, Hao Y, Singh RP. Biofortification strategies to increase grain zinc and iron concentrations in wheat. Journal of Cereal Science. 2014; **59**(3):365-372. DOI: 10.1016/j.jcs.2013.09.001

[35] Clemens S. Zn and Fe biofortification: The right chemical environment for human bioavailability. Plant Science. 2014;**225**:52-57. DOI: 10.1016/j.plantsci.2014.05.014

[36] Vasconcelos MW, Gruissem W, Bhullar NK. Iron biofortification in the 21st century: setting realistic targets, overcoming obstacles and new strategies for healthy nutrition. Current Opinion in Biotechnology. 2017;**44**:8-15. DOI: 10.1016/j.copbio.2016.10.001

[37] Lv C, Zhao G, Lönnerdal B. Bioavailability of iron from plant and animal ferritins. The Journal of Nutritional Biochemistry. 2015;**26**(5):532-540. DOI: 10.1016/j.jnutbio.2014.12.006

Chapter 5

Heart Failure and Iron Deficiency

Francesco Fedele, Alessandra Cinque,
Massimo Mancone, Viviana Maestrini and
Carmen Caira

Additional information is available at the end of the chapter

http://dx.doi.org/10.5772/intechopen.79358

Abstract

Heart failure (HF) is a major public health problem because it is one of the most common causes of morbidity and mortality in Western countries, with a prevalence of 1–2% in the adult population, rising to ≥10% in those age >70 years. In addition to the "classic" co-morbidities, such as COPD, arterial hypertension, diabetes, renal failure, etc., there are other conditions frequently found in patients with heart failure that many times are underestimated. One example are anemia and iron deficiency (ID). ID, regardless of anemia impair exercise tolerance, symptoms and quality of life, with a strong negative prognostic impact on hospitalization and mortality rate. Despite strong evidence of high prevalence of ID in these patients and current guidelines recommendations, the diagnosis of ID and its monitoring over time still have low priority for physicians in clinical practice. Consequently ID is under-treated; furthermore current therapies, in particular i.v. iron as ferric carboxymaltose, though effective, turn out to be poorly managed by clinicians. ID should be considered more in real world HF healthcare settings to improve patients' quality of life and outcome.

Keywords: heart failure, heart disease, anemia, iron deficiency

1. Heart failure and comorbidity

Heart failure (HF) is a major public health problem because it is one of the most common causes of morbidity and mortality in Western countries, with a prevalence of 1–2% in the adult population, rising to ≥10% in those age >70 years [1]. Regardless of the cause, HF is a life threatening syndrome and therefore requires specific treatments aimed at reducing symptoms and improving quality and/or quantity of life. The overall aging of the population,

IntechOpen

© 2018 The Author(s). Licensee IntechOpen. This chapter is distributed under the terms of the Creative Commons Attribution License (http://creativecommons.org/licenses/by/3.0), which permits unrestricted use, distribution, and reproduction in any medium, provided the original work is properly cited. (cc) BY

that has been recorded over the last few decades, has led to an increase in the prevalence of chronic pathologies, from which derives an increase in the number of elderly people that have more than one disease at the same time. Patients with HF have multiple co-morbid conditions and 60% of them have five or more [2, 3]. In addition to the "classic" co-morbidities, such as COPD, arterial hypertension, diabetes, renal failure, etc., there are other conditions frequently found in patients with heart failure that many times are underestimated. One example are anemia and iron deficiency (ID): the presence of ID, regardless of concomitant anemia, has been shown to worsen symptoms and patient prognosis.

Management of co-morbidities is a key point of HF patients care, to cut down this chronic epidemic disabling syndrome.

2. Iron deficiency in heart failure

2.1. Epidemiology

Iron deficiency (ID) is a frequent co-morbidity found in 35–50% of patients with HF; it is the most common cause of anemia in patients with HF but, most importantly, ID occurs in 46% of non-anemic patients with stable systolic HF [4, 5].

Despite its high prevalence, this co-morbidity was underdiagnosed for several years. ID can be present in patients with HF regardless of the presence of anemia and can be classified in absolute or functional ID, by determining ferritin levels: ferritin <100 μg/l if absolute ID, reflecting depleted iron stores due to low dietary intake, blood loss, etc., or ferritin between 100 and 300 μg/l and the transferrin saturation (<20%) if functional ID, when iron delivery to target cells is impaired despite normal or overly abundant iron stores, due to chronic inflammation, etc. [6, 7].

ID in chronic HF is more frequent in women and in patients with advanced HF, as shown by Klip data [4]: in an international cohort of 1506 patients with chronic HF, ID was closely related to disease severity, assessed using NYHA functional class (**Figure 1**) and NT-proBNP levels.

ID frequently overlaps with anemia and chronic kidney disease; in this study only the 7% of patients had anemia without ID (related to renal dysfunction, hemodilution, vitamins or folic deficiency, hematologic cause) [8–10].

As reported in a study of Ponikowski, ID prevalence was of 37% in a cohort of 546 CHF patients (32 ± 4 vs. 57 ± 10% in subjects without vs. with anemia) [11]. This study also showed that ID, but not anemia, was related to an increased risk of mortality after 3 years follow-up (**Figure 2**).

In the setting of acute heart failure patients, ID prevalence is even higher (50–80%) [12, 13].

In preserved ejection fraction HF it is also high, as showed in subgroups analysis.

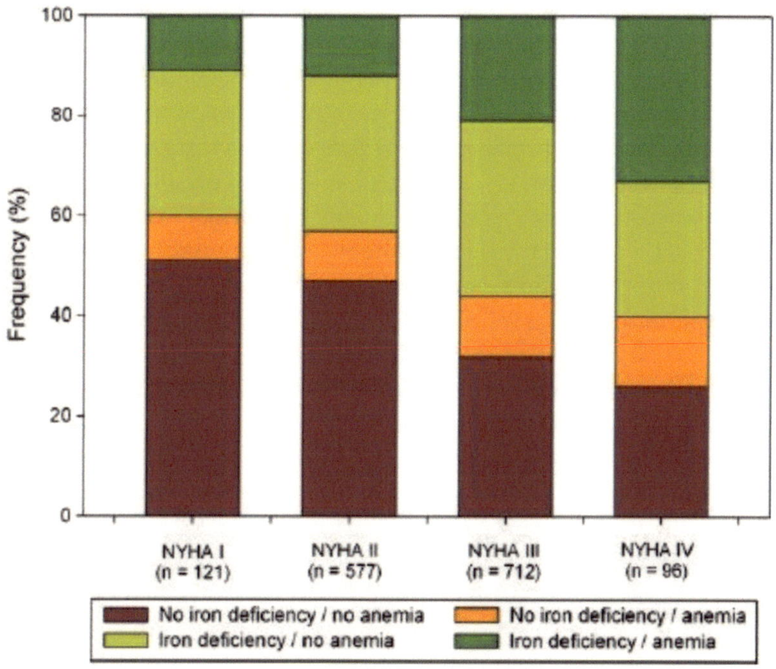

Figure 1. ID and anemia stratified by NYHA functional class. Modify by Iron deficiency in chronic heart failure: an international pooled analysis.

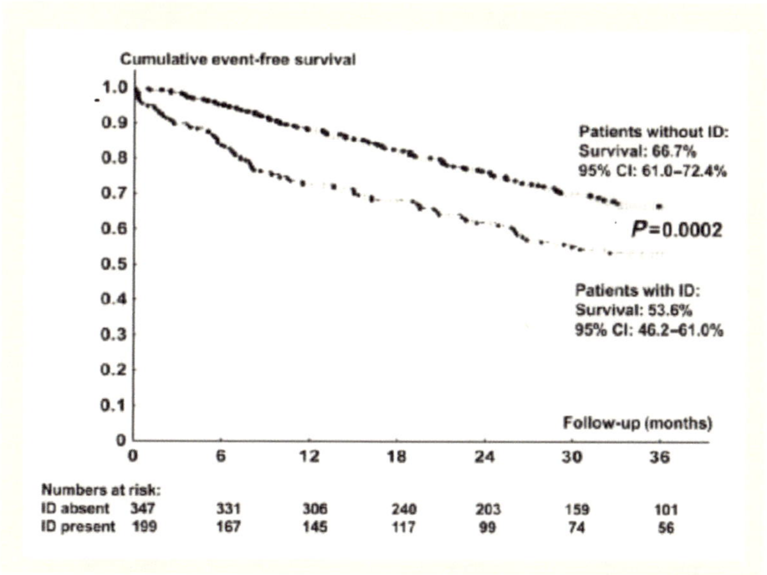

Figure 2. ID was related to an increased risk of mortality after 3 years follow-up. Modify by Iron deficiency: an ominous sign in patients with systolic chronic heart failure.

2.2. Clinical and prognostic impact

In patients with chronic HF, ID, regardless of the presence of anemia, is a strong and independent predictor of outcome, in fact it is associated with higher mortality and hospitalization rates [13, 14]. Moreover, ID has been shown to worsen HF symptoms and to impair exercise tolerance, with poor quality of life [11]. The explanation is simple and is related to the key role of iron in human homeostasis. Iron, as is well known, is essential for erythropoiesis, as part of the hemoglobin, ad so for oxygen transport. Moreover, as is perhaps less well known [15], iron is a fundamental co-factor for other several processes, such as normal activity of key enzymes of the citric acid cycle and ROS scavenging enzymes. It plays an important role in generation of ATP, necessary for all cellular process and for muscles contractility. Recent in vitro evidence show that ID directly affects human cardiomyocytes function, impairing mitochondrial respiration, and reducing contractility and relaxation. In this regard, a special characteristic of physical stress in heart failure is the early shift from aerobic to anaerobic metabolism due to the compromission of oxidative capacity [16]. It is therefore clear that ID can only worse exercise intolerance and sub-maximal exercise resistance, heavily compromising quality of life. Restoration of intracellular iron levels can reverse these effects [17]. Exercise tolerance was analyzed in 443 patients with systolic chronic heart failure: only ID (and not anemia) was significantly associated with reduced peak oxygen consumption (VO_2) (**Figure 3**) [18].

Another study from Okonko confirm these data on 157 chronic HF patients: ID was related to impaired exercise capacity and survival and appeared prognostically more ominous than anemia [19]. In the same way, it is known that ID therefore has a negative impact on Quality

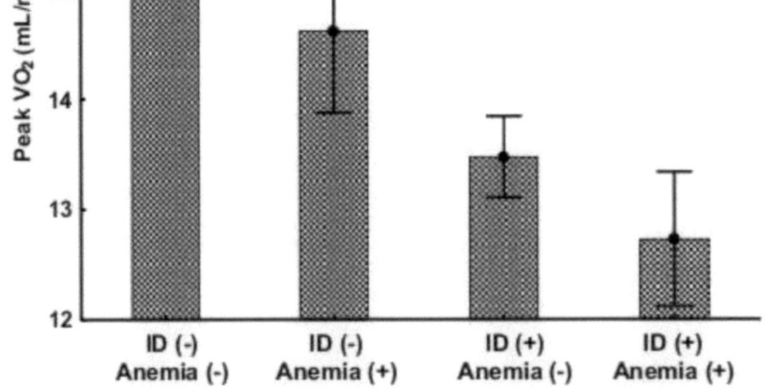

Figure 3. ID is significantly associated with reduced peak VO_2. Modify by Iron deficiency predicts impaired exercise capacity in patients with systolic chronic heart failure.

of Life, measured by Minnesota Living with Heart Failure questionnaire, and this is independent of the presence of anemia. Lower TSAT is related to lower QoL; the correlation is not so clear for hemoglobin level [20]. Furthermore, ID is a strong and independent predictor of outcome in HF patients, as shown in several studies. In the large international pooled cohort of 1506 chronic HF patients by Klip, ID identifies those with an enhanced risk for death, independently of other well-established predictors of outcome, and appears to have greater predictive power than anemia (**Figures 4** and **5**) [4].

For several years, we consider only anemia as negative prognostic factor, but definitely, the negative effect of iron deficiency seems to be stronger.

2.3. Treatments

Given the clinical importance of ID in HF patients, restoration of iron stores to normal levels should be a therapeutic goal in clinical practice [21], as well as addressing its underlying causes.

Regardless the known poor efficacy, oral iron supplementation is almost always the first line therapy for ID, due to their low cost and ease of administration. Ferrous sulfate is the most commonly used. However, gastrointestinal side effects are common and can often compromise the therapy compliance. Moreover, the enteric absorption may be reduced by quite a lot of factors: interaction with other drugs or food, edema and congestion of the gastrointestinal mucosa, high hepcidin level in HF [22].

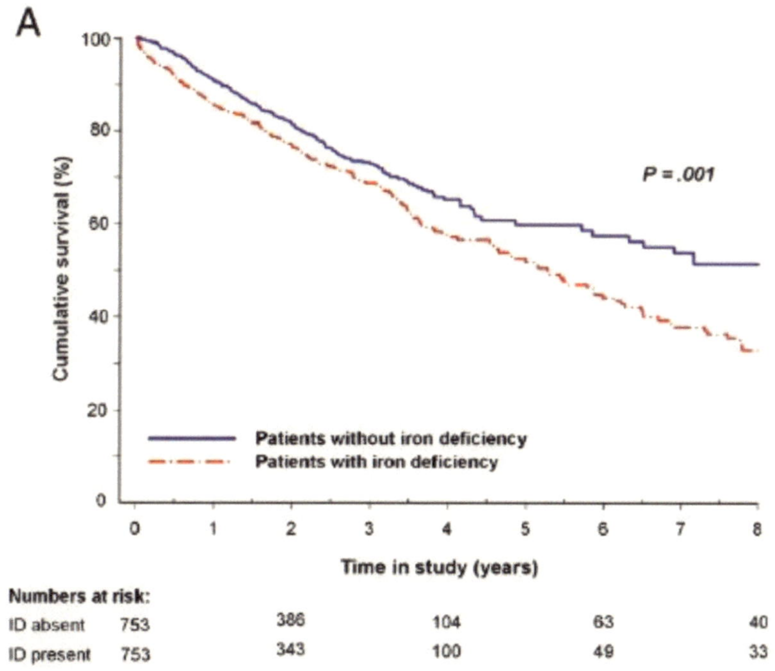

Figure 4. ID is a strong and independent predictor of outcome in HF patients. Modify by Iron deficiency in chronic heart failure: an international pooled analysis.

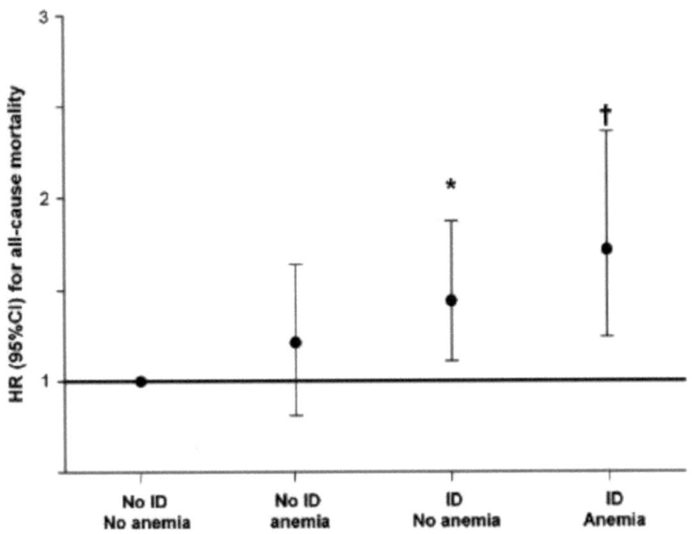

Figure 5. Mortality among groups of ID and/or anemia (* p<0.01; † p<0.001). Modify by Iron deficiency in chronic heart failure: an international pooled analysis.

In addition, iron deficiency in HF patients is severe in the most of the case (on average 1.5–2 g of iron); considering that a tablet has 80 mg of iron (with a bioavailability of 10%), the supplement must be prolonged for months to be effective. As we will see later, the use of iron salt is not supported by clinical trials data.

Intravenous iron may solve these problems and may be more suitable both for physicians and patients [23, 24]. Intravenous iron complex used for ID are ferric gluconate, ferric carboxymaltose, ferric hydroxide sucrose, and ferric hydroxide dextran. A big advantage of intravenous iron is the rapid improvement in iron parameters [25]: it is not influenced by hepcidin absorption blocking mechanisms. Probably it is also cost-effectiveness, because reduce hospitalization and improved quality of life [26].

Comparative data from the different complex are not available. However, ferric carboxymaltose has the advantage of high dose (500 mg) formulation [27]: it seems to be particularly effective in severe ID, that is frequently diagnosed in HF patients, and well tolerated. One or two injections are usually adequate to reach the therapeutic target.

The most of clinical trials on ID correction in HF evaluated the use of ferric carboxymaltose.

2.4. From clinical trials to guidelines

The FAIR-HF study was the first big multicentric, prospective, double-blind, randomized trial [28] published in the contest of iron supplementation in HF, almost 10 years ago. Patients were randomized to receive intravenous ferric carboxymaltose or placebo. Quality of life, symptoms, distance during 6-minute walking test were significantly improved after treatment with ferric carboxymaltose in patients with chronic HF and ID, with or without anemia. A such strong result was really not expected. The clinical improvement was confirmed in several patient's subgroups, based on hemoglobin level, renal function, gender, ejection fraction. Moreover, intravenous iron improved patient's global assessment and NYHA class in both anemic and non-anemic patients with HF.

Another trial, CONFIRM-HF [11], was performed in heart failure patients with iron deficiency. It was a multicentre, double-blind, placebo-controlled trial that enrolled 304 ambulatory symptomatic HF patients with left ventricular ejection fraction ≤45%, elevated natriuretic peptides, and iron deficiency. The primary endpoint was the exercise capacity. Ferric carboxymaltose significantly improved 6 minutes walking test distance from baseline to week 24. Moreover the treatment may be associated with risk reduction of hospitalization for worsening HF at week 52; although it was a secondary endpoint, it had an amazing relevance.

The EFFECT-HF trial was a multicenter, randomized 1:1, open label, standard of care controlled trial [29]; the primary endpoint was change in peak VO_2 from baseline to week 24. Again, intravenous ferric carboxymaltose significantly improve exercise capacity in heart failure patients. The main limit of this trial was that standard of care not include intravenous iron, but just oral formulation.

So, treatment with intravenous ferric carboxymaltose in patients with HF and iron deficiency improves iron stores.

Whether ferric carboxymaltose seems to be associated with an improved clinical condition and outcome in these high-risk patients, further study are necessary.

In the last few months was performed an individual patient meta-analysis on the topic [30]. Individual patient data were extracted from randomized clinical trials comparing ferric carboxymaltose with placebo in patients with systolic HF and ID. The endpoints were recurrent cardiovascular hospitalizations and cardiovascular mortality. About 839 patients, of whom 504 were randomized to FCM, were included. Ferric carboxymaltose was associated with a reduction in cardiovascular hospitalizations.

The results of this analysis show that treatment of ID with e.v. ferric carboxymaltose in ambulatory systolic HF patients with ID may decrease recurrent cardiovascular hospitalizations.

These findings suggest that intravenous iron therapy may potentially represent a beneficial addition to the standard medical management of HF (**Table 1**).

Although the individual patient meta-analysis is the best type of statistical analysis, a specific randomized clinical trial is needed.

About oral iron therapy, the most relevant trial published is the IRONOUT trial [31]. It was a double-blind, placebo-controlled randomized clinical trial of patients with reduced ejection fraction (<40%). Oral iron polysaccharide (150 mg twice daily) was compared to placebo. Among patients with HF with iron deficiency, high-dose oral iron did not improve exercise capacity over 16 weeks and did not change iron biomarkers. Probably the absorption from

Recurrent event outcomes	FCM (N = 504)	Placebo (N = 335)	p
	NB. Total events (incidence per 100 patient-years of follow-up)		
CV hospitalization and CV death	69 (23.0)	92 (40.9)	0.009
HF hospitalization and CV death	39 (13.0)	60 (26.7)	0.011
CV hospitalization and all-cause death	71 (23.7)	94 (41.8)	0.009
HF hospitalization and all-cause death	41 (13.7)	62 (27.6)	0.011
All-cause hospitalization and all-cause death	108 (36.1)	118 (52.5)	0.060
HF hospitalization	22 (7.3)	43 (19.1)	0.003
CV hospitalization	52 (17.4)	75 (33.3)	0.004
All-cause hospitalization	89 (29.7)	99 (44.0)	0.056

Modify by Effects of ferric carboxymaltose on hospitalizations and mortality rates in iron-deficient heart failure patients: an individual patient data meta-analysis.

Table 1. Results from individual patient meta-analysis by Anker et al.

the gastrointestinal tract is limited by foods, medications, edema of the intestinal mucosa due to venous congestion [32], upregulation of hepcidin [33]. Moreover, each tablet has a dose of iron that is very low (compared with the massive iron deficiency that affects heart failure patients), so the treatment should be prolonged for several months. These results do not support use of oral iron supplementation in patients with HfrEF.

Based on the actual evidence, the current ESC guidelines on diagnosis and treatment of HF [1] recommend very clearly that all patients with HF have to be screened for ID based on serum ferritin and TSAT (Class I, Level C) (**Figure 6**). The dosage of ferritin and TSAT has the same strong of recommendation of the evaluation of hemoglobin and white cells, sodium, potassium, urea, creatinine, glucose, liver function test and other routine analysis. We also have the specific recommendation regarding the treatment: intravenous ferric carboxymaltose should be considered in symptomatic patients with HFrEF and iron deficiency in order to alleviate HF symptoms, and improve exercise capacity and quality of life (**Figure 7**). It is important to note that when the guidelines were published there was not available the results of meta-analysis from Anker that showed the benefits in terms of heart failure hospitalization and cardiovascular death.

Based on the results of FAIR-HF and CONFIRM-HF trials, the 2017 ACC/AHA/HAS guidelines for management of HF [34, 35] also state that IV iron might be reasonable in NYHA Class II to III patients with ID (Class II, Level B) to improve QoL and functional status.

2.5. Real world data

In addition to clinical trials and guidelines, real world data confirm not only the high prevalence and the negative prognostic impact of ID in HF patients, but also the efficacy of i.v. iron, in particular of FCM, to treat this important comorbidity. But, despite this background, real world data show also what is still happening today in clinical practice, that is the poor attention paid to the diagnosis and treatment of ID in HF patients.

Recommendations	Class[a]	Level[b]
The following diagnostic tests are recommended/should be considered for initial assessment of a patient with newly diagnosed HF in order to evaluate the patient's suitability for particular therapies, to detect reversible/treatable causes of HF and co-morbidities interfering with HF:		
- haemoglobin and WBC - sodium, potassium, urea, creatinine (with estimated GFR) - liver function tests (bilirubin, AST, ALT, GGTP) - glucose, HbA1c - lipid profile - TSH - ferritin, TSAT = TIBC	I	C
- natriuretic peptides	IIa	C

Figure 6. Recommendations for diagnostics tests in patients with heart failure. Modify by ESC HF guidelines.

Recommendations	Class[a]	Level[b]	Ref[c]
Iron deficiency			
Intravenous FCM should be considered in symptomatic patients with HFrEF and iron deficiency (serum ferritin <100 μg/L, or ferritin between 100–299 μg/L and transferrin saturation <20%) in order to alleviate HF symptoms, and improve exercise capacity and quality of life.	IIa	A	469, 470

Figure 7. Recommendations for the treatment of other comorbidities in patients with heart failure. Modify by ESC HF guidelines.

The PReP prospective Registry [36] show that in a real world setting of 1198 ambulatory patient with HF, ID was present in 42.5% of the study participants, and not previously known in any of them. The prevalence of anemia was 18.9%, and it was known prior to enrolment only in 4.8% of participants. ID, more common in anemic patients, was an independent predictor of reduced exercise tolerance. The authors conclude that despite high prevalence and clinical relevance, ID and anemia are often unappreciated in real world ambulatory HF patients.

Regarding treatment, although several Clinical trials studied FCM use and efficacy, real world evidence is limited. Nunes data [37] show that in 459 HF outpatient with ID treated with FCM therapy, Hb and TSAT increased and FCM was well tolerated; moreover higher doses of FCM (500 mg–1000 mg and 100-3000 mg) showed a significant higher efficacy compared with lower dose (500 mg).

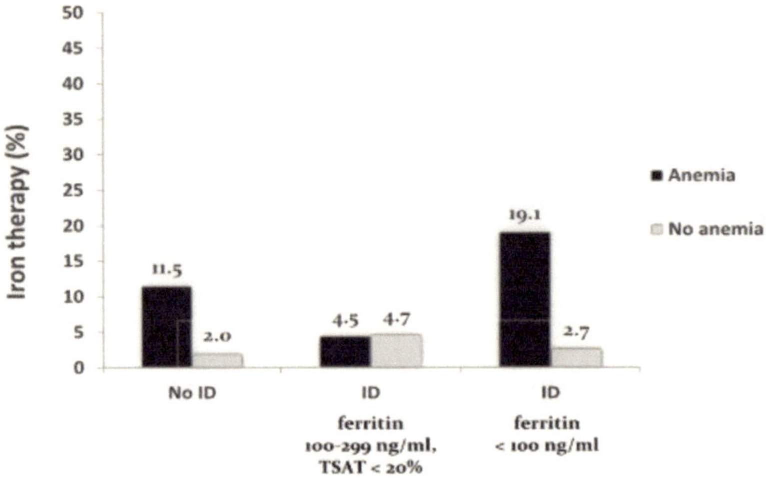

Figure 8. ID is under-treated, especially in non-anemic patients. Modify by RAID-HF registry.

But, despite these data, current guidelines and the results of IRONOUT trial, in real world oral iron is often the first line therapy for ID in HF, that remain an underdiagnosed comorbidity as showed by Wienbergen in the sub-study of the RAID-HF registry [38], aimed to obtain information on ID management in a large real world cohort of HF patients. The results showed that among 1484 participants, iron status was determined only in 62% of them (and 55% had ID), despite it was a registry focusing on ID in HF! Furthermore only 8.5% of ID patients received iron therapy, most of them orally and just 11 of the 13 patients treated with i.v. iron received FCM. Patients on iron therapy had higher NYHA class and were predominantly anemic; physicians analyzed and treated ID only in severe HF or in presence of anemia (**Figure 8**); and it is not evidence based because the efficacy of iron therapy is demonstrated independently of anemia.

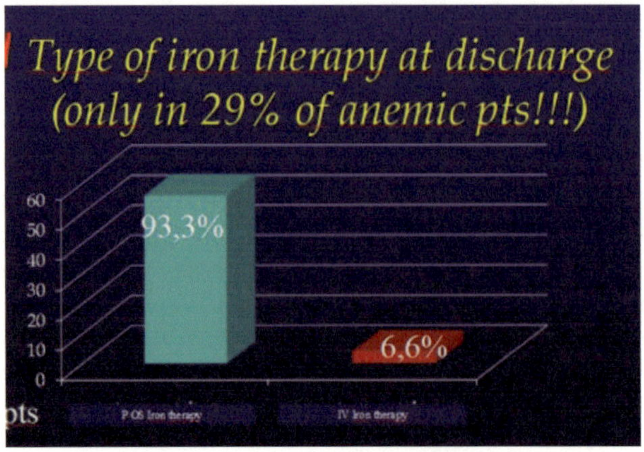

Figure 9. Type of iron therapy at discharge. Modify by Carmes-1 study.

These real word data, that confirm the results of our CARMES 1 study in a cohort of 418 hospitalized HF patients in Italy in which ID was underdiagnosed and undertreated [39] (**Figure 9**), underline that diagnostic and therapeutic efforts on ID management in HF are still low in clinical practice.

3. Conclusion

Iron deficiency, regardless of anemia, is a frequent co-morbidity in HF patients, which impair exercise tolerance, symptoms and quality of life, with a strong negative prognostic impact on hospitalization and mortality rate.

Despite strong evidence of high prevalence of ID in these patients and current guidelines recommendations, the diagnosis of ID and its monitoring over time still have low priority for physicians in clinical practice. Consequently ID is under-treated; furthermore current therapies, in particular i.v. iron as FCM, though effective, turn out to be poorly managed by clinicians.

Therefore ID should be considered more in real world HF healthcare settings to improve patients' quality of life and outcome.

Author details

Francesco Fedele[1]*, Alessandra Cinque[1], Massimo Mancone[1], Viviana Maestrini[1] and Carmen Caira[2]

*Address all correspondence to: francesco.fedele@uniroma1.it

1 Department of Cardiovascular, Respiratory, Nephrologic and Anesthesiologic Sciences, Sapienza University of Rome, Rome, Italy

2 Sacra Famiglia Hospital – Fatebenefratelli. Erba, Como, Italy

References

[1] Ponikowski P, Voors AA, Anker SD, Bueno H, Cleland JGF, Coats AJS, Falk V, Gonzalez-Juanatey JR, Harjola VP, Jankowska EA, Jessup M, Linde C, Nihoyannopoulos P, Parissis JT, Pieske B, Riley JP, Rosano GMC, Ruilope LM, Ruschitzka F, Rutten FH, van der Meer P. 2016 ESC guidelines for the diagnosis and treatment of acute and chronic heart failure. European Heart Journal. 2016;**37**:2129-2200

[2] Wong CY, Chaudhry SI, Desai MM, Krumholz HM. Trends in comorbidity, disability, and polypharmacy in heart failure. The American Journal of Medicine. Feb 2011;**124**(2): 136-143

[3] Nakano H, Toshiyuki N, Varum S, Michikazu N, Kunihiro N, Yasuyuki H, Satoshi H, Naotsugu I, Yasuo S, Yasuhide A, Takeshi A, Teruo N, Kengo K, Hiroyuki Y, Hisao O, Satoshi Y, Tashiro C, Toshihisa A, on behalf of the Na DEF Investigators. Impact of iron deficiency on long term clinical outcomes of hospitalized patients with heart failure. International Journal of Cardiology. 2018;**261**:114-118

[4] Klip IT, Comin-Colet J, Voors AA, Ponikowski P, Enjuanes C, Banasiak W, Lok DJ, Rosentryt P, Torrens A, Polonski L, van Veldhuisen DJ, van der Meer P, Jankowska EA. Iron deficiency in chronic heart failure: An international pooled analysis. American Heart Journal. Apr 2013;**165**(4):575-582

[5] Doehner W, Blankenberg S, Erdmann E, Ertl G, Hasenfuß G, Landmesser U, Pieske B, Schieffer B, Schunkert H, von Haehling S, Zeiher A, Anker SD. Iron deficiency in chronic heart failure: Diagnostic algorithm and present-day therapeutic options. Deutsche Medizinische Wochenschrift. May 2017;**142**(10):752-757

[6] Wish JB. Assessing iron status: Beyond serum ferritin and transferrin saturation. Clinical Journal of the American Society of Nephrology. Sep 2006;**1**(Suppl 1):S4-S8

[7] Dignass A, Farrag K, Stein J. Limitations of serum ferritin in diagnosing Iron deficiency in inflammatory conditions. International Journal of Chronic Diseases. Mar 18, 2018;**2018**:9394060. DOI: 10.1155/2018/9394060 eCollection 2018

[8] Nanas JN, Matsouka C, Karageorgopoulos D, Leonti A, Tsolakis E, Drakos SG, Tsagalou EP, Maroulidis GD, Alexopoulos GP, Kanakakis JE, Anastasiou-Nana MI. Etiology of anemia in patients with advanced heart failure. Journal of the American College of Cardiology. Dec 19, 2006;**48**(12):2485-2489

[9] Solomakhina NI, Nakhodnova ES, Ershov VI, Belenkov YN. The role of hepcidin in formation of anemia of chronic disease and iron deficiency anemia in elderly and old patients with chronic heart failure. Kardiologiia. Mar 2018;**3**:20-27

[10] Cunha GJL, Rocha BML, Menezes Falcão L. Iron deficiency in chronic and acute heart failure: A contemporary review on intertwined conditions. European Journal of Internal Medicine. Jun 2018;**52**:1-7

[11] Jankowska EA, Rozentryt P, Witkowska A, Nowak J, Hartmann O, Ponikowska B, Borodulin-Nadzieja L, Banasiak W, Polonski L, Filippatos G, McMurray JJ, Anker SD, Ponikowski P. Iron deficiency: An ominous sign in patients with systolic chronic heart failure. European Heart Journal. Aug 2010;**31**(15):1872-1880

[12] Cohen-Solal A, Damy T, Terbah M, Kerebel S, Baguet JP, Hanon O, Zannad F, Laperche T, Leclercq C, Concas V, Duvillié L, Darné B, Anker S, Mebazaa A. High prevalence of iron deficiency in patients with acute decompensated heart failure. European Journal of Heart Failure. Sep 2014;**16**(9):984-991

[13] Nunez J, Comin-Colet J, Minana G, Nunez E, Santas E, Mollar A, Valero E, Garcia-Blas S, Cardells I, Bodi V, Chorro FJ, Sanchis J. Iron deficiency and risk of early readmission following a hospitalization for acute heart failure. European Journal of Heart Failure. Jul 2016;**18**(7):798-802

[14] Nakano H, Nagai T, Sundaram V, Nakai M, Nishimura K, Honda Y, Honda S, Iwakami N, Sugano Y, Asaumi Y, Aiba T, Noguchi T, Kusano K, Yokoyama H, Ogawa H, Yasuda S, Chikamori T, Anzai T, NaDEF Investigators. Impact of iron deficiency on long-term clinical outcomes of hospitalized patients with heart failure. International Journal of Cardiology. Jun 15, 2018;**261**:114-118

[15] Rocha BML, Cunha GJL, Menezes Falcão LF. The Burden of Iron Deficiency in Heart Failure: Therapeutic Approach. Journal of the American College of Cardiology. 2018 Feb 20;**71**(7):782-793

[16] Martens P, Verbrugge FH, Nijst P, Dupont M, Mullens W. Limited contractile reserve contributes to poor peak exercise capacity in iron-deficient heart failure. European Journal of Heart Failure. Apr 2018;**20**(4):806-808

[17] Hoes MF, Grote Beverborg N, Kijlstra JD, Kuipers J, Swinkels DW, Giepmans BNG, Rodenburg RJ, van Veldhuisen DJ, de Boer RA, van der Meer P. Iron deficiency impairs contractility of human cardiomyocytes through decreased mitochondrial function. European Journal of Heart Failure. May 2018;**20**(5):910-919

[18] Jankowska EA, Rozentryt P, Witkowska A. Iron deficiency predicts impaired exercise capacity in patients with systolic chronic heart failure. Journal of Cardiac Failure. 2011;**17**:899-906

[19] Okonko DO, Mandal AKJ, Missouris CG, Poole-Wilson PA. Disordered iron homeostasis in chronic heart failure. Journal of the American College of Cardiology. Sep 2011; **58**(12):1241-1251

[20] Enjuanes C, Klip IT, Bruguera J, Cladellas M, Ponikowski P, Banasiak W, van Veldhuisen DJ, van der Meer P, Jankowska EA, Comín-Colet J. Iron deficiency and health-related quality of life in chronic heart failure: Results from a multicenter European study. International Journal of Cardiology. Jun 15, 2014;**174**(2):268-275

[21] McDonagh T, Macdougall IC. Iron therapy for the treatment of iron deficiency in chronic heart failure: Intravenous or oral? European Journal of Heart Failure. Mar 2015;**17**(3):248-262

[22] Jankowska EA, von Haehling S, Anker SD, Macdougall IC, Ponikowski P. Iron deficiency and heart failure: Diagnostic dilemmas and therapeutic perspectives. European Heart Journal. Mar 2013;**34**(11):816-829

[23] Jankowska EA, Drozd M, Ponikowski P. Iron deficiency treatment in patients with heart failure. Handbook of Experimental Pharmacology. 2017;**243**:561-576

[24] Gstrein C, Meyer M, Anabitarte P. Iron substitution in the treatment of chronic heart failure. Swiss Medical Weekly. Jul 11, 2017;**100**:w14453

[25] Ponikowski P, van Veldhuisen DJ, Comin-Colet J, Ertl G, Komajda M, Mareev V, McDonagh T, Parkhomenko A, Tavazzi L, Levesque V, Mori C, Roubert B, Filippatos G, Ruschitzka F, Anker SD. CONFIRM-HF investigators. Beneficial effects of long-term

intravenous iron therapy with ferric carboxymaltose in patients with symptomatic heart failure and iron deficiency. European Heart Journal. Mar 14, 2015;**36**(11):657-668

[26] Hofmarcher T, Borg S. Cost-effectiveness analysis of ferric carboxymaltose in iron-deficient patients with chronic heart failure in Sweden. Journal of Medical Economics. 2015;**18**(7):492-501

[27] Scott LJ. Ferric carboxymaltose: A review in iron deficiency. Drugs. Mar 2018;**78**(4):479-493

[28] Anker SD, Comin Colet J, Filippatos G, Willenheimer R, Dickstein K, Drexler H, Luscher TF, Bart B, Banasiak W, Niegowska J, Kirwan BA, Mori C, von Eisenhart Rothe B, Pocock SJ, Poole-Wilson PA, Ponikowski P. FAIR-HF trial investigators. Ferric carboxymaltose in patients with heart failure and iron deficiency. The New England Journal of Medicine. Dec 17, 2009;**361**(25):2436-2448

[29] van Veldhuisen DJ, Ponikowski P, van der Meer P, Metra M, Böhm M, Doletsky A, Voors AA, Macdougall IC, Anker SD, Roubert B, Zakin L, Cohen-Solal A. Effect of ferric carboxymaltose on exercise capacity in patients with chronic heart failure and Iron deficiency. Circulation. Oct 10, 2017;**136**(15):1374-1383

[30] Anker SD, Kirwan BA, van Veldhuisen DJ, Filippatos G, Comin-Colet J, Ruschitzka F, Lüscher TF, Arutyunov GP, Motro M, Mori C, Roubert B, Pocock SJ, Ponikowski P. Effects of ferric carboxymaltose on hospitalizations and mortality rates in iron-deficient heart failure patients: An individual patient data meta-analysis. European Journal of Heart Failure. 2018;**20**:125-133

[31] Lewis GD, Malhotra R, Hernandez AF, McNulty SE, Smith A, Felker GM, Tang WHW, LaRue SJ, Redfield MM, Semigran MJ, Givertz MM, Van Buren P, Whellan D, Anstrom KJ, Shah MR, Desvigne-Nickens P, Butler J, Braunwald E. Effect of oral iron repletion on exercise capacity in patients with heart failure with reduced ejection fraction and iron deficiency: The IRONOUT HF randomized clinical trial. Journal of the American Medical Association. May 16, 2017;**317**(19):1958-1966

[32] Sandek A, Bjarnason I, Volk HD, Crane R, Meddings JB, Niebauer J, Kalra PR, Buhner S, Herrmann R, Springer J, Doehner W, von Haehling S, Anker SD, Rauchhaus M. Studies on bacterial endotoxin and intestinal absorption function in patients with chronic heart failure. International Journal of Cardiology. 2012;**157**:80-85

[33] Niehaus ED, Malhotra R, Cocca-Spofford D, Semigran M, Lewis GD. Repletion of iron stores with the use of oral iron supplementation in patients with systolic heart failure. Journal of Cardiac Failure. Aug 2015;**21**(8):694-697

[34] Yancy CW, Jessup M, Bozkurt B, Butler J, Casey DE, Colvin MM, Drazner MH, Filippatos GS, Fonarow GC, Givertz MM, Hollenberg SM, Lindenfeld J, Masoudi FA, McBride PE, Peterson PN, Stevenson LW, Westlake C. 2017 ACC/AHA/HFSA focused update of the 2013 ACCF/AHA guideline for the management of heart failure: A report of the American College of Cardiology/American Heart Association Task Force on Clinical Practice Guidelines and the Heart Failure Society of America. Journal of Cardiac Failure. Aug 2017;**23**(8):628-651

[35] Bozkurt B. What is new in heart failure management in 2017? Update on ACC/AHA heart failure guidelines. Current Cardiology Reports. Apr 17, 2018;**20**(6):39

[36] Von Haehling S, Gremmler U, Krumm M, Mibach F, Schön N, Taggeselle J, Dahm JB, Angermann CE. Prevalence and clinical impact of iron deficiency and anaemia among outpatients with chronic heart failure: The PrEP registry. Clinical Research in Cardiology. Jun 2017;**106**(6):436-443

[37] Nunes AR, Fonseca C, Marques F, Belo A, Brilhante D, Cortez J. Prevalence of anemia and iron deficiency in older Portuguese adults: An EMPIRE substudy. Geriatrics & Gerontology International. 2017;**17**:1814-1822

[38] Wienbergen H, Pfister O, Hochadel M, Michel S, Bruder O, Remppis BA, Maeder MT, Strasser R, von Scheidt W, Pauschinger M, Senges J, Hambrecht R. Usefulness of iron deficiency correction in management of patients with heart failure [from the registry analysis of iron deficiency-heart failure (RAID-HF) registry]. The American Journal of Cardiology. Dec 15, 2016;**118**(12):1875-1880

[39] Caira C, Ansalone G, Mancone M, Canali E, Pagliaro M, Fratarcangeli L, Aznaran CA, Gatto MC, Di Pietro R, Fedele F. Heart failure and iron deficiency anemia in Italy: Results from CARMES-1 registry. Future Cardiology. May 2013;**9**(3):437-444

Chapter 6

Neurocognitive Dysfunctions in Iron Deficiency Patients

Elena Zhukovskaya, Alexander Karelin and Alexander Rumyantsev

Additional information is available at the end of the chapter

http://dx.doi.org/10.5772/intechopen.82620

Abstract

In this chapter, the authors described the actuality of the investigations of neurocognitive dysfunctions in patients with iron deficiency. In infants, the incidence of iron deficiency is 73%; the probability of its transition to iron deficiency anemia is very high. The development of myelin at an early age reduces the production of myelin, and the formation of g-aminobutyric acid worsens the metabolism of dopamine in the striatal brain, which leads to slowing of motor function and behavioral problems in the child. Children with iron deficiency conditions are prone to developmental delays, reduced school performance, and behavioral disorders. In older adults, cognitive dysfunctions depend on complications of the vascular nature, complicated by comorbid iron deficiency. Concomitant pathology also influences iron homeostasis. The regulating mechanisms of iron deficiency, as the same cognitive deficiency, despite the age involve more than 200 proteins from iron homeostasis, appropriate cofactors: derivatives of vitamin B, copper, manganese, zinc ions, enzymes, cell growth factors, etc. All these partners could influence separately or together to the development of iron deficiency and a complication of it neurocognitive dysfunctions. The combination of iron deficiency anemia and iron deficiency with comorbid pathology often exacerbates cognitive problems and requires a weighted approach to the choice of therapeutic correction tactics.

Keywords: iron deficiency, neurocognitive dysfunction, comorbid pathology, iron homeostasis

IntechOpen

© 2019 The Author(s). Licensee IntechOpen. This chapter is distributed under the terms of the Creative Commons Attribution License (http://creativecommons.org/licenses/by/3.0), which permits unrestricted use, distribution, and reproduction in any medium, provided the original work is properly cited.

1. Introduction

Iron deficiency (ID) and iron deficiency anemia (IDA) could have multifocal pathologic effects [1–3]. However, one of the most socially significant consequences of ID is the burden to the cognitive abilities of the population [4–6]. At present, the prevalence of iron deficiency and iron deficiency anemia is 2–6% among European children. Given the importance of iron deficiency relative to proper cognitive development and the alterations that can persist through adulthood because of this deficiency, the objective of this study was to review the current state of knowledge about this health problem [7]. In fact, there is a consensus that ID, without, concurrent anemia, has the same negative impact on cognition, behavior, and motor skills that can persist in the long-term [8]. So, the verification of ID in young age can be particularly important, because of the influence on the mental health and further cognitive functions during the whole life of the people [9–11].

Neurophysiologic methodologies are noninvasive approaches that can provide information about the functional integration of the CNS [12, 13]. For example, dramatic decreases in latencies in auditory and visual evoked potentials in infancy are often used to index the overall intactness and maturation of the CNS. Progressively, shorter latencies, until adult levels are achieved, are thought to reflect the increasing speed of transmission through sensory pathways, resulting in large part from increased myelination of the auditory and optic nerves and at the intracerebral level [14, 15].

Pathophysiological mechanisms of unfavorable impact on nervous system started in utero [16, 17]. The essential factors modifying the ID neurotoxicity are its depth and duration [18, 19]. Evidence suggests that neonatal Fe status may be compromised as a consequence of maternal ID [20, 21]. Genes, infections, malnutrition, and other factors affecting fetal brain development are a major component of risk for a child's emotional development and later mental illnesses, including schizophrenia, bipolar disorder, and autism [22–25]. As part of comprehensive maternal and fetal care, prenatal nutrient interventions should be further considered as uniquely effective first steps in decreasing risk for future mental illnesses and cognitive dysfunctions in newborn children [26–28]. Moreover, this fact makes the study of cognitive impairments in ID states especially urgent, because in recent years, the survival of preterm newborns has increased. Many of them have problems with iron deficiency. Every year in France, almost 35,000 babies (4–4.5%) are born at 35–36 weeks, 13,000 (1.5%) at 32–34 weeks, and 13,000 (1.5%) at less than 32 weeks (i.e., very preterm) [29]. In 2008, deliveries at 32–33, 34–36, and 37–38 weeks accounted for 1.2, 7.5, and 29.7%, respectively, of all births in the United States. Currently, depth preterm infants born at 32–33 weeks gestation and infants born at 34–36 weeks gestation make up the largest subgroup of preterm infants and contributors to more than 80% of premature births in the United States [30]. Multiple births currently account for nearly 3.5% of all births in the United States [31]. The health of neonates born to women carrying multiple fetuses is of concern, as this group alone is responsible for 15% of all preterm births and 20% of all low birth weight infants born in the United States [32]. More than 110,000 newborns in Russia are preterm [33].

IDA and ID often develop in children and adults with other diseases that lead to impaired cognitive functions. Moreover, in such a situation, intellectual dysfunctions are formed because of the action of several pathophysiological mechanisms. Feinstein in 1970 had introduced the concept of comorbidity, defining it as the presence of a separate additional clinical episode that exists or can manifest itself against the background of the current disease and always differs from it [34]. In addition, the introduction of perinatal factors, a number of concomitant diseases (comorbid diseases) occur in a person at different periods of his life [35, 36].

Obesity and ID are two of the most common nutritional disorders in the world. In children, both conditions deserve particular attention. ID and obesity have been independently associated with poor cognitive function, but now the pathophysiological mechanism(s) linking obesity, ID, and cognitive dysfunction is unknown. Questions related to neuronal effects of insulin remain largely controversial. However, in the last decade, convincing evidence has been obtained that insulin and insulin-receptor signaling the brain system is necessary for normal functioning neurons [37]. Dysfunction of this system leads to the development of neurodegenerative diseases [38–40]. The interaction between ID and obesity in determining cognitive dysfunction could be driven by elevated hepcidin and reduced iron bioavailability in obese children. Pediatricians should bear in mind the potential effect of obesity-related ID on cognition in obese children and the need to evaluate both iron status and the presence of cognitive dysfunction [41, 42].

When considering the position of "iron as a victim" in obesity, emphasis is placed on mechanisms that cause sideropenia, as well as the accumulation of iron in adipose tissue. It is assumed that from this moment, the story "iron as a suspect" begins in the pathogenesis of obesity. There is a possibility of forming a vicious circle, in which ID, cumulating of iron in adipose tissue and direct obesity, is self-sustaining processes [43]. Several studies revealed an association between obesity and ID in children and, in some cases, a reduced response to oral supplementation of iron [44]. Randomized trials of low-dose iron supplementation (≤60 mg daily) for pregnant women are warranting testing the relationship between iron oxidative stress and insulin resistance/gestational diabetes, especially for iron-replete women. The connecting mechanism, however, is not completely known. This review is focused on the following: ID in obese children and the role of hepcidin in the connection between body fat and poor iron status; iron status and consequences on health, in particular on cognitive function; cognitive function and obesity; suggestion of a possible link between cognitive dysfunction and ID in pediatric obesity; and implications for therapy and future research [45].

There are a vast number of conditions affecting iron metabolism in all age groups [46–48]. Some of this leads to the appearance of ID, for example, with acute hemorrhage or chronic pathology. Recent studies addressing the physiological effects of poor iron status on physical performance, including work productivity, voluntary activity, and athletic performance in postmenopausal women are addressed. Similarly, the effects of iron status on neurological performance, including cognition, effect, and behavior, are observed [49]. Cognitive impairment is common in elderly heart failure patients and is independently associated with anemia and renal dysfunction. Further studies are needed to assess whether optimal treatment of anemia and chronic kidney disease may prevent the development of cognitive impairment in heart failure patients [50].

ID was identified as a risk factor regarding the severity of several symptoms even without low hemoglobin level among chronic hemodialysis patients, and supplementation of iron was considered efficacious for improving critical symptoms affecting those undergoing maintenance dialysis [51].

Normally, timely recovery of the required number of red blood cells leads to rapid compensation of the patient's condition, but adverse effects of IDA or ID could influence insufficient cognitive function in many acute and chronic diseases in adults [52].

The primary pathological mechanism of the concomitant diseases is hypoxemia of the brain tissue, stress-mediated vascular reactions, chronic inflammation in obesity, etc. [53–55]. Common causes of absolute ID in heart failure patients are drug interactions, poor dietary iron intake, gastrointestinal malabsorption, and gastrointestinal blood loss [56–59]. ID is a frequent comorbidity in preserved ejection fraction and is associated with reduced exercise capacity and quality of life. Its prevalence increases with increasing severity of diastolic dysfunction [60]. Anemia in elderly patients with concomitant atherosclerosis and arterial hypotension is a significant risk factor for transient ischemic attacks and ischemic stroke, and diabetes is the adverse impact for cognitive abilities. IDA and subcortical ischemic change might be associated with increased risks for cognitive impairment among the elderly [61, 62].

At the current stages of science, many problems of synergy between ID and comorbid diseases for cognitive functions in patients have not been resolved, which makes it challenging to choose effective therapy.

2. Neurocognitive dysfunctions

The Latin term "cognitio"—the functioning of human cognition, more precisely, is the ability to understand the ongoing process. Tolman first proposed the formulation in 1948 [63]. Cognition began to be studied not only in philosophy but also in the specific sciences—psychology, physiology, medicine, pedagogy, etc. [64, 65]. Cognitive functions are perception, ingenuity, the ability to get acquainted with new information and memorize it, attention, speech, orientation in space and time, and motor skills. In children with ID, cognitive impairments lead to a delay in intellectual development, difficulties in educating. Based on the fact that neurons are the morphological substratum for cognitive functions, scientists often use the term neurocognitive. However, the most base evidence data were achieved in children population. The initial status of children could be determined by the results of complex clinical and psychological diagnosis, which are aimed at assessing the cognitive and motor spheres. The panels of the tests to diagnose the neurocognitive and motor dysfunctions in children and adults include numerous tests, widely used in current medicine [66, 67].

Examples of the tests to diagnose neurocognitive dysfunctions:

1. Visual selective reminding TOMAL samples of various domains of memory in children and adolescents, ages 5 years 0 months through 19 years 11 months, 30 days. The TOMAL is composed of a core battery of 10 subtests, including 5 verbal and 5 nonverbal subtests, as well as supplementary subtests (3 verbal and 1 nonverbal). Four TOMAL subtests assess retrieval both immediately upon stimulus presentation and following a 30-min filled

delay. Among the 10 core subtests, memory for stories involves immediate and delayed free recall of short verbal narratives and word selective reminding is a verbal list learning task that includes a delayed free recall condition [68].

2. First proposed by Swiss psychologist André Rey in 1941 and further standardized by Paul-Alexandre Osterrieth in 1944, it is frequently used to further explain any secondary effect of brain injury in neurological patients, to test for the presence of dementia, or to study the degree of cognitive development in children. The "Rey– Alexander Osterrieth complex figure test" (ROCF) is a neuropsychological assessment in which examinees are asking to reproduce a complicated line drawing, on the first copy it freehand (recognition), and then drawing from memory (recall) [69]. Many different cognitive abilities are needed for a correct performance, and the test, therefore, permits the evaluation of different functions, such as visuospatial abilities, memory, attention, planning, and working memory (executive functions) [70].

3. Verbal fluency tests are semantic verbal fluency tests with the categories Animals and Fruit and could be used for lexical/phonemic ability versions due to the educational heterogeneity of the local population, which sometimes limits the use of instruments that require knowledge acquired through higher formal education [71].

4. Visual-motor integration is using the Beery-Buktenica Developmental Test of Visual-Motor Integration (Beery VMI) (Beery, 1989; Beery, 1996; Beery and Beery, 2004). The Beery VMI is comprised of drawings of geometric forms that increase in difficulty. The forms are copied with paper and pencil and scored based on objective scoring criteria outlined in the test manuals according to how accurately they were copied when compared to the original. The Beery VMI has been demonstrating good reliability and validity as reported in the manual [72, 73].

5. The "Bruninx-Ozeretskii test" was estimate using for motor function of the person. The child is asked to perform a series of game tasks available for understanding children from 4 years. The person is given a clear instruction describing the nature of the task, and then the researcher shows the child an image on the cardboard a card showing a child performing the same task. With difficulties in perception of the patient information, the researcher, as an example, performs the task itself and then invites the child to repeat it. The result is integrated into the indicator "General motor rating", presenting in the form of a percentile scale with the maximum and minimum values from 20 to 80. The Achenbach System of Empirically Based Assessment, created by Thomas Achenbach [74, 75], is a collection of questionnaires used to assess adaptive and maladaptive behavior and overall functioning in individuals. The system includes report forms for multiple informants—the Child Behavior Checklist is used for caregivers to fill out ratings of their child's behavior; the Youth Self Report Form (YSR) is used for children to rate their own behavior; and the Teacher Report Form is used for teachers to rate their pupil's behavior. The ASEBA seeks to capture consistencies or variations in behavior across different situations and with different interaction partners [76].

6. IntegNeuroTM is standardized and semiautomated computerized battery assesses sensorimotor function, attention, new learning and memory, language fluency, executive

function, and estimated intelligence. A total of 50 healthy individuals were included in the study. Correlational analyses revealed highly significant associations between the two cognitive batteries. These results support the use of IntegNeuroTM as a computerized cognitive system. Additional studies are needed to examine the clinical utility of the battery [77].

This tests and/or other could be used not only at the baseline but also for monitoring neurocognitive dysfunctions.

3. Iron deficiency and nervous system

The concentration of iron in the brain reaches 21.3 mg per 100 mg, whereas in the liver—only 13.4 mg per 100 mg. Iron serves as a critical cofactor for proteins involved in a host of biological processes. Iron is of central importance to many vital processes because the metal is a catalytic component of crucial metabolic enzymes in the citric acid cycle, mitochondrial respiration, replication, or neurotransmitter synthesis [78]. Synapse growth is examined specifically in conditions of iron deficiency in the Drosophila. It is shown that projections of the small ventrolateral clock neurons to the protocerebrum of the adult Drosophila brain are significantly reduced upon chelation of iron from the diet. This growth defect persists even when iron is restored to the diet. Genetic neuronal knockdown of ferritin 1 or ferritin 2, critical components of iron storage and transport, does not affect synapse growth in these cells. Together, these data indicate that dietary iron is necessary for central brain synapse formation in the fly and further validate the use of this model to study the function of iron homeostasis on brain development [79–81].

In the monkey model, scientists show that both during and after a period of ID, iron-dependent neural processes are affected, which raises the potential concern that the anemia commonly experienced by many growing infants that could have a protracted effect on the developing brain. To further investigate the effects of ID on the immature brain, 49 infant rhesus monkeys were evaluated across the first year of life. The mothers, and subsequently the infants after weaning, were maintained on a standardized diet containing 180 mg/kg of iron and were not provided other iron-rich foods as treats or supplements. As the infants grew, they were all screened with hematological tests, which documented that 16 (33.3%) became markedly ID between 4 and 8 months of age. During this anemic period and subsequently at 1 year of age, cerebrospinal fluid (CSF) specimens were collected to compare monoamine activity in the ID and iron-sufficient infants. Monoamine neurotransmitters and metabolite levels were normal at 4 and 8 months of age, but by 1 year, the formerly anemic monkeys had significantly lower dopamine and significantly higher norepinephrine levels. These findings indicate that ID can affect the developmental trajectory of these two important neurotransmitter systems, which are associated with emotionality and behavioral performance, and further that the impact on the young monkey was most evident during the period of recovery [82].

ID in the first year of life can have a negative impact on the processes of postnatal central nervous system (CNS) formation, which can have long-term consequences for the development

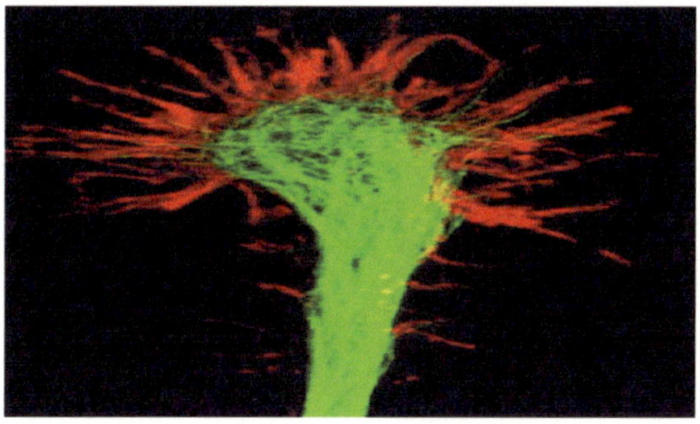

Figure 1. Growth cone of axon (https://www.turkaramamotoru.com/ru/).

of the child [83]. Several decades ago, it was believed that new brain cells in an adult are not formed. That person can study only up to 25 years, and then the brain has lost the chance to be educated. Those intellectual abilities are inherited or inherent in quality, and they cannot be developed during the life. Now we know that this is not so. The human brain develops all his life (**Figure 1**). In the world literature, the influence of ID and IDA on the functioning of the human and animal organism, including on the nervous system is discussed [81, 84].

By the time of birth, the baby's brain is immature. Nevertheless, with each month the child learns more and more. To make the signals go quickly and in the right direction, the nerve fibers in an adult person are isolated. Just like electrical wires. A substance that performs the role of isolation is called a myelin or myelin sheath. Nerve cells maintain a connection with each other with the help of processes, which are called dendrites and axons or nerve fibers [85, 86]. Signals on these fibers almost instantly move from cell to cell. It is like how electricity flows through the wires (**Figure 2**). Genes control myelination. To activate them, the cells of the brain need iron. ID inhibits myelination, as it does not allow cells to maintain high activity of these genes. Therefore, children with ID can develop hyperactivity and lack of attention in the future. From the fact that myelin is in lack, the nervous system will not learn to isolate and direct the signals well [87].

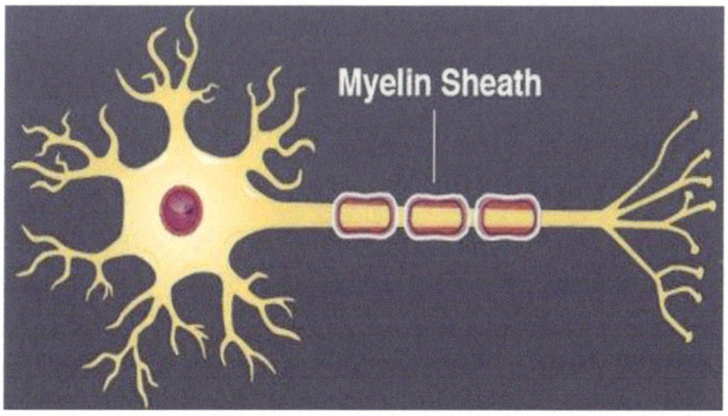

Figure 2. Location of myelin sheath in neuron (https://www.goconqr.com/en-US/p/615525).

Iron homeostasis impairment is also a component of peripheral neuropathies [88]. The main function of the peripheral nervous system (PNS) is to collect impulses from the periphery and transfer them to the CNS, where they are integrated to generate an adequate response. PNS neurons extend over a significant length that in humans can reach above 1 m in extension [89]. Thus, a correct and fast conduction of electrical impulses is essential for rapid and maximal response. In vertebrates, this is achieved by the generation of myelin [90]. Besides providing axonal insulation, several evidences indicate that myelin is essential also for neuronal protection. In the absence of myelin, axons degenerate, and this is the main cause of morbidity in demyelinating and demyelinating disorders. The homeostasis of iron in the PNS influence, on its transport across the blood-nerve barrier, its involvement in myelination [16].

Restless legs syndrome is one of the examples of peripheral neuropathies. The pathophysiology of idiopathic restless legs syndrome is still incompletely understood; however, it is well established that disturbances of dopaminergic function and alterations of iron homeostasis are involved in its pathogenesis [91–93]. Concerning iron metabolism, the general hypothesis is that iron deficiency is common in RLS patients, as reflected by reduced iron levels in brain sections, measurements of decreased iron levels in the cerebrospinal fluid, and imaging studies indicating iron dyshomeostasis in the brain [94].

The quality and quantity of sleep are increasingly recognized as important factors in human development, with concomitant effects on affective behavior and cognitive performance [95]. In addition to biological mechanisms, cultural factors are also important determinants of sleep practices and behaviors in infants, children, and adolescents, and influence both the type and frequency of sleep problems found in the pediatric population [96]. IDA in infancy is associated with long-lasting neurofunctional effects despite iron treatment; the normal development of sleep patterns might be affecting. Night polysomnographic recordings were performed in 55 healthy 4-year-old children (former IDA = 27 and nonanemic controls = 28). Both groups were followed from infancy and were similar in background characteristics. The duration of each waking episode was measured, as was the duration of each episode of no rapid eye movement (NREM) sleep stages 1 (NREM1), 2 (NREM2), and 3–4 (SWS), and rapid eye movement (REM) sleep. The data were analyzed according to the successive thirds of the total sleep time (TST). Relative to controls, former IDA children showed: (a) longer duration of REM sleep episodes in the first third and shorter in the last third, (b) more REM sleep episodes in the first third and fewer in the second third, and (c) shorter latency to the first REM sleep episode and shorter NREM stage 2 and SWS episodes within the first sleep cycle. The results show that early IDA is associated with long-lasting alterations in the temporal organization of sleep patterns [97, 98].

The work reveals CNS developmental delay through the study of qEEG (less rapid and slower frequencies) which recovered significantly with iron supplementation. It is concluded that IDA constitutes a high risk factor for a lag of CNS maturation [99]. Neuroscientists who use MRI in a special functional mode also found activation of whole areas of the brain during their use. And they also saw "holes" in the activity of the brain, in those people, which lead an unhealthy lifestyle or get micronutrients: iron, other trace elements, and vitamins [94]. Genes also control neuroplasticity. Iron is necessary for their activation. Fetal-neonatal iron deficiency dysregulated genes important for hippocampal development both acutely and persistently into early adulthood [100, 101]. A number of studies have shown that cognitive functions, especially memory in women with iron deficiency, are reduced compared with their peers without deficiency. In other words, their brains do not have enough resources to train. However, unlike myelination, active neuroplasticity is not limited in time, but occurs throughout life [102].

The rate of development of the nervous system of the child also slows down with ID [103]. For complex skills, extensive neural networks are needed. To have neural networks, myelin is needed. If it is not enough, new skills are late. This is most noticeable in speech. Children with latent ID or anemia in their first year of life usually start talking later. Evoked potentials provide noninvasive measures of nerve transmission and CNS functioning. Auditory brainstem responses and visual evoked potentials show dramatic changes in infancy, largely as a result of progressive myelination. Because iron is required for normal myelination, pathway transmission in these sensory systems is affected by early iron deficiency. Absolute latencies for all auditory brainstem responses and visual evoked were significantly longer in former IDA children [104, 105].

Some studies have established that cognitive impairment may be closely associated with neuroanatomical damage and zinc metabolism in the hippocampus due to iron deficiency, which may result from abnormal cholinergic function. The hippocampus is the focus of many studies today, since this brain structure has high zinc concentration and is highly involved in many forms of cognitive deficits as a consequence of cholinergic deficiency and has achieved prominence because of dementia in aging and Alzheimer's disease [106]. Thus, it is now apparent that cognitive impairment may not be attributed to a single neurotransmitter, but rather, alterations and interactions of several systems in different brain regions. In animal models of iron deficiency, it is apparent that dopaminergic interaction with the opiate system and cholinergic neurotransmission may be defective [107].

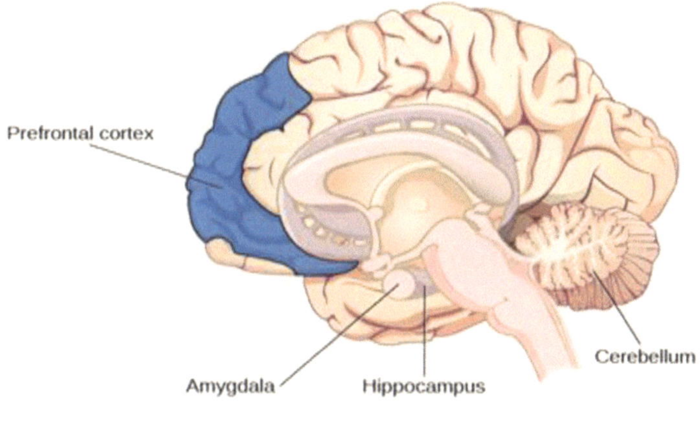

Figure 3. The location of hippocampus (http://www.thinglink.com/scene/834791711828869120).

Memory can also suffer from lack of iron in early childhood. The hippocampus is the region of the brain responsible for memory. It forms, stores, and reproduces the knowledge and experience of a person. The quality of memory and the speed of reproduction depend on the development of neural networks of the hippocampus. The main parts of the brain involved with memory are the amygdala, the hippocampus, the cerebellum, and the prefrontal cortex (**Figure 3**).

Studying the effect of iron deficiency on the hippocampus of laboratory animals, scientists discovered an interesting fact. In rats suffering from iron deficiency in utero, the hippocampus at birth is less in volume than in their peers, with which the gland lacked. Moreover, these changes persist when rats grow [108, 109]. It is assumed that the human iron deficiency affects the hippocampus in a similar way [110]. In addition, it is assumed that changes in dopamine metabolism in the brain occur in response to ID, as well as altered serotonergic neurotransmission and dopamine receptor function [7, 111].

Chronic ID during development, independent of anemia, alters the adult mouse hippocampal transcriptome. Restoring iron status during a known critical period of hippocampal neurodevelopment incompletely normalized these changes, suggesting a need for additional studies to identify the most effective timeline for iron therapy and adjunctive treatments that can fully restore ID-induced molecular changes, particularly in human populations in whom chronic ID is endemic [112].

The problem of attention deficit hyperactivity disorder (ADHD) is actually everywhere. Different international groups confirmed the correlation of iron serum parameters, serum ferritin, and ADHD. Indian pediatricians with a high level of significant found that serum ferritin level was significantly lower among ADHD patients. This finding is consistent with multiple previous studies [113, 114]. Many other studies reported an association between iron deficiency and ADHD [115, 116].

Based on the stroke registry at the Hospital for Sick Children (Toronto, Ontario, Canada), physicians found that comparatively previously healthy children with stroke were 10 times more likely to have IDA than healthy children without stroke. Furthermore, children with iron deficiency anemia accounted for more than half of all stroke cases in children without an underlying medical illness, which suggests that iron deficiency anemia is a significant risk factor for stroke in otherwise healthy young children. Primary prevention and early identification of iron deficiency anemia must remain a priority [117].

4. Iron deficiency and cognition

In fact, patients with chronic ID are presented with lower grades in the language, perception of ambient sound, and motor measures compared with children with normal dietary iron status [118, 119]. Moreover, Lozoff et al., the most productive researcher of this term, reported that changes in the mesolimbic pathway, positive influence, and inherent reward could support the explanation of the altered social-emotional behavior described in children with ID. Thus, the status of iron appears to be the decisive determinant of cognitive functioning in children, and its destruction implies significant consequences for the health of the child. Improvement of iron status in 12-months and 6-years children has diminished the public health threat associated with iron depletion in the population studied [120]. Therefore, actions to prevent iron depletion in infancy remains are very important [121, 122].

The infant period of life with ID dramatically influence at the intellectual functions. Iron deficiency in first year of life occurs at a time point of rapid neural development and when morphological, biochemical, and bioenergetics alterations take place. The structures of the brain can either become abnormal because of ID in utero or in early postnatal life because iron is essential for proper neurogenesis and differentiation of certain brain cells and brain regions [123, 124]. Early ID alters the transcriptome, metabolome, structure, intracellular signaling pathways, and electrophysiology of the developing hippocampus, the brain region responsible for recognition learning and memory. Until recently, it was unclear whether these effects are directly due to lack of iron interacting with important transcriptional, translational, or post-translational processes or to indirect effects such as hypoxia due to anemia or stress [125].

Data indicate poorer object permanence and short-term memory encoding and/or retrieval in infants with IDA at 9 months. These cognitive effects were attributable, in part, to IDA-related deficits in socioemotional function. Children with poor socioemotional performance seem to be more vulnerable to the effects of IDA on cognitive function IDA [126, 127]. Improved iron status at 12 months and 6 years has diminished the public health threat associated with iron depletion in the population studied [128].

Several previous studies have shown that children with low levels of iron in their blood do worse than those who without ID on tests that measure cognitive skills, such as thinking, learning, and memory, according to the background information in the article [129]. Researches from the University of Michigan studied the long-term effects of ID and socioeconomic status in a group of 185 children from an urban area in Costa Rica. The children, who were an average of 17 months old when the study began in 1983–1985, were screened for ID at their first visit. They were given cognitive tests (on which the index, or overall average score, is 100) then and again at ages 5, 11–14, 15–18, and 19 years. Those who had low iron levels in infancy even after 3 months of iron therapy were compared with those who had normal iron levels either without or after treatment. The gap in cognitive scores between iron-deficient and non-ID teens had widened to 25 points (70.4 vs. 95.3). "The observed pattern appears to make sense in terms of the cumulative and transactional nature of cognitive development." Acquisition of new skills is intimately linked to mastery of skills at an earlier developmental level. If direct and indirect effects of early ID on the brain disrupted or delayed basic developmental processes, there could be a snowball effect. In an economically stressed family environment, there might not be the resources or capacity to help children compensate. The authors conclude that the results highlight the necessity to identify the children at risk for ID and prevent or treat the condition in infancy [130].

Rates of ID are high among healthy young women. Cognitive impairment occurs secondary to ID in infants and children, but evaluation of the impact on cognition among young women is inconsistent. The aim of the research was to determine the suitability of the IntegNeuro test battery for assessing cognitive function in ID and iron-sufficient young women. A pilot double-blinded, placebo-controlled intervention trial was conducted in iron-deficient (serum ferritin ≤20 μg/L and hemoglobin >120 g/L) and iron-sufficient young women (18–35 years). Cognitive function and hematological markers of iron status were measured at baseline and follow-up. Iron-deficient participants (n = 24) were randomized to receive placebo, 60 or 80 mg elemental iron daily supplements for 16 weeks. A control group of iron-sufficient participants (n = 8) was allocated to placebo. Change scores for impulsivity and attention were significantly greater in plasma ferritin improvers than in nonimprovers (p = 0.004, p = 0.026). IntegNeuro was easy to administer and acceptable to young women. Based on the differences in memory and attention scores between iron-deficient participants on iron treatment and those on placebo, it was decided that between 26 and 84 participants would be required in each iron treatment group for an adequately powered extension of this pilot study [131].

In Archangelsk, Russia ID without iron deficiency anemia was diagnosed in 46.7% of the children among 90 children aged 7–8 years attending comprehensive schools. Contingency of Toulouse-Piéron test results with the level of serum iron was evaluated by means of Pearson $\chi2$-test, the effect being determined by "phi" coefficient. Statistically significant association was detected between the level of serum iron and AIP of Toulouse-Piéron test ($\chi2 = 21.878$ and $p = 0.039$) with a relatively strong effect ($\varphi = 0.493$). The study has shown that ID without IDA has a negative effect on the accuracy of information processing [132].

ID and, in an even greater degree, IDA affects the formation of such a complex psychosocial effect as social isolation [133]. The consequences of this phenomenon during schooling can restrain the realization of the child's cognitive abilities. Children who are iron deficient (ID) or iron-deficient anemic (IDA) have been shown to seek and receive less stimulation from their caregivers, contributing to functional isolation. Over time, the reduced interactions between child and caregiver are thought to interfere with the acquisition of normative social competencies and adversely affect the child's development [31].

5. Deficiency of iron in patients with imbalance of micronutrients

Numerous vitamins, macro- and microelements, indispensable components, and nutrition of a person represent the value of the micronutrient complex, since they are necessary for the occurrence of numerous biochemical reactions in the body, including ensuring human intellectual abilities. Micronutrients are chemically and physiologically active substances that are able to interact with other substances, as well as with each other. These interactions can lead to an increase or decrease in the effect of taking vitamin-mineral complexes. For example, calcium and zinc reduce the absorption of iron. Moreover, the addition of vitamins A, C, and others—strengthen, contributing to the correction of IDA and ID.

A frequent cause of neurocognitive impairment is a mono or poly-micronutrient deficiency. The micronutrient deficiency mostly delivers during pregnancy [134, 135]. For an example widespread iron deficiency, iodine deficiency is a monodeficiency, that is, are due to a lack of only one element. Iron is the most abundant transition metal in biology and an essential cofactor for many cellular enzymes. The literature on the effects of micronutrients on cognitive, motor, and behavioral development is reviewed focusing mainly on children. Iron, zinc, iodine, and vitamins are discussed. The review is selective and concentrates on the more recent work and areas of controversy. There are well-established associations with poor development and iron and iodine deficiencies but the deficiencies usually occur in disadvantaged circumstances, and establishing causal relationships is difficult [136]. More than 200 proteins of iron homeostasis cannot function without corresponding cofactors: derivatives of group B vitamins, copper ions, manganese, zinc, etc. [137, 138]. For example, 9 copper-containing enzymes and 22 manganese-dependent proteins are involved in the homeostasis of iron.

In addition to iron, microelements such as copper and cobalt, to a lesser extent manganese, zinc, etc., play an important role in the processes of normal development of nervous system. According to the National Nutrition Monitoring Bureau of India, IDA is diagnosed in many healthy children, and two-thirds have clinical symptoms of ID combined with a deficiency of essential trace elements such as iodine, zinc, copper, etc. [139]. Hypermanganesemia in children with SLC39A14 gene mutation (OMIM 608736 8p21.3) is associated with severe ID [140].

Copper is an immediate participant in the transfer of elemental iron to the bone marrow and the formation of mature forms of erythrocytes from their precursors—reticulocytes; it promotes the utilization of iron for the formation of hemoglobin molecules. Physiological variables of iron and copper are related to each other [141]. One of the key enzymes of the "respiratory chain" of electron transfer is cytochrome C oxidase, containing a copper and iron ion as cofactors. Therefore, copper can be considered one of the main synergists of iron [142].

Fe(II) and Cu(II) act synergistically to delay anaerobic growth of bacteria environmentally relevant metal concentrations [143]. The lack of copper also leads to the exhaustion of the nervous system. The deficiency in the activity of Cu, Zn-superoxide dismutase due to genetic defects, and deficiencies in zinc or copper leads to amyotrophic lateral sclerosis, a neurodegenerative disease of motor neurons. In addition to influence the processes of inflammation, the activity of superoxide dismutase affects the hemolysis of erythrocytes and the cellular homeostasis of iron [144]. There are other works determining the place of combined trace elements in the pathogenesis of neurodegenerative diseases [145].

Supplementation studies in infants and elder children revealed that zinc might also play a major role in brain function based on strong evidence from experimental animals. Zinc deficiency gestation in mice, rats, and rhesus monkeys caused impaired learning, reduced attention, and poor memory in their offspring. There is lack of data in humans and inconclusive. With respect to brain function alone, other nutrients such as docosahexaenoic acid (DHA, 22:6 n-3 fatty acid) improve visual acuity and mental development in small-for-gestational-age infants, folate supplementation during pregnancy prevents neural tube defect in infants, and selenium deficiency in animals affects activities of brain enzymes necessary for brain development and function [146, 147]. Critical issues to be considered include: single versus multiple limiting nutrients, critical period of deficiency, responsive indicators and variables that may affect the results as environmental, and psychological and social factors [148, 149].

Studies of trace element deficiency in the children's population of the Chelyabinsk region, carried out in 2014, confirmed the widespread occurrence of ID conditions. More than 40%

of adolescents aged 13–15 years had misbalances of essential trace elements. The most often deficiency of iron was associated with lack of copper, zinc, chromium, phosphorus, and magnesium. Deficiency of iron was more pronouncing against the background of increased content of heavy metals in biosubstrates: hair and blood of the adolescents surveyed [150].

Vitamin D deficiency was also associated with moderate anemia among young children. The role of vitamin D, vitamin B-12, and folic acid in risk for anemia in multi-nutrient deficiency responsible for cognitive development needs to be examined in further studies [151–154].

5.1. The role of erythropoietin in cognitive dysfunctions

Since 1906, thanks to the pioneering work of French scientists, R. Carnot and S. Deflandre, erythropoietin (EPO) has become known primarily as a hemopoietin factor stimulating the formation of red blood cells de novo. They found that after bleeding a rabbit, there was, in its serum 24 h later, some factor which stimulated red cell production in normal rabbits. They called it hemopoietin, but it was later called erythropoietin [155].

EPO (**Figure 4**) is an important renal hormone, and the secretion of which is regulated by such factors as the blood supply of the kidneys, the level of iron in the blood plasma, the cross hormonal effects from the sympathetic nervous system, and endocrine glands [50, 156]. Recently, it became known that EPO, in spite of its name, is important not only for the regulation of erythropoiesis but also for the regulation of the growth and multiplication of cells of a number of other tissues, including, importantly, the cells of the nervous system. Thus, EPO is an important growth factor for neurons [157, 158].

The authors demonstrate with the animal model that EPO would diminish the deleterious effects of a social stressor in mice. Indeed, EPO induced anxiolytic and antidepressant-like responses in a forced swim test, open field, elevated-plus maze, and a novelty test and appeared to blunt some of the negative behavioral effects of a social stressor. Furthermore, EPO promoted adult hippocampal neurogenesis, an important feature of effective antidepressants. The EPO could be recommended as a possible adjunct treatment for affective disorders, as well as other stressor-associated disorders of impaired neuroplasticity [159, 160].

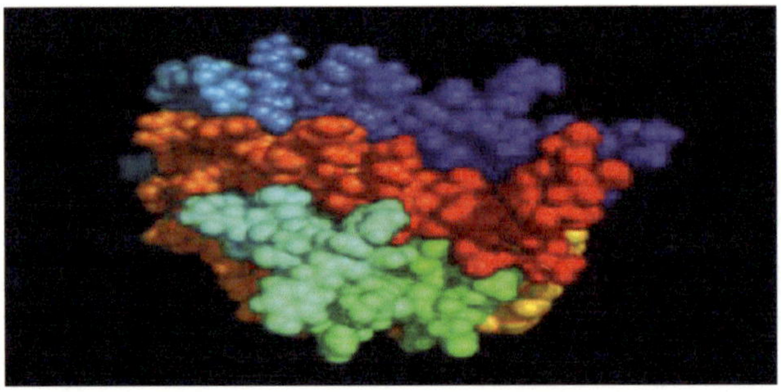

Figure 4. The structure of the erythropoietin molecule (http://en.turkcewiki.org/wiki/Erythropoiesis-stimulating_agent).

EPO, which is widely prescribed to treat anemia, has recently emerged as a potent neurotrophic factor with robust actions on the brain. A slight decrease in the level of EPO is also observed in patients with depressed states not suffering from chronic renal failure, in part because, as it turned out in recent years, the brain is also one of the places of EPO secretion, where it plays the role of a neuropeptide. EPO receptors are found in areas of the brain important for cognitive functioning, such as the hippocampus and the prefrontal cortex. One of the important reasons for the development of depression and cognitive impairment in chronic renal failure patients is the reduction in the secretion of EPO by the kidneys. The introduction of recombinant human EPO in patients with CRF improves their overall well-being, cognitive function and reduces the level of depression regardless of the effectiveness of treatment with erythropoietin anemia [161]. It has been shown that the administration of recombinant human EPO-alpha or beta has an antidepressant effect and improves the cognitive function of patients with depression, even those who do not suffer from renal failure [162, 163]. It is also interesting to note that the most effective antidepressant treatment/electroconvulsive therapy is accompanied by a marked increase in the secretion of EPO by brain tissue. It has also been shown that the additional administration of exogenous EPO can not only enhance the antidepressant effect of electroconvulsive therapy but also reduce the cognitive impairment caused by electroconvulsive therapy [164, 165].

In one of the first prospectively designed studies IDA, evaluation of the better neurocognitive outcomes was found of preterm infants randomized to receive Darbepoetin (Darbe) in compared with placebo. Preterm infants had significantly higher cognitive scores compared with the placebo group. Authors reported decreased transfusions and donor exposures in preterm infants randomized to Darbe or EPO compared with placebo. As these erythropoiesis-stimulating agents (ESA) have shown promise as neuroprotective agents. Of the original 102 infants (946 ± 196 g and 27.7 ± 1.8 weeks' gestation), 80 (29 EPO, 27 Darbe, and 24 placebo) returned for follow-up. The three groups were comparable for age at testing, birth weight, and gestational age. After adjustment for gender, the analysis of covariance revealed significantly higher cognitive scores among Darbe (96.2 ± 7.3; mean ± SD) and EPO recipients (97.9 ± 14.3) compared with placebo recipients (88.7 ± 13.5; $P = .01$ vs. ESA recipients) as was object permanence ($P = .05$). No ESA recipients had cerebral palsy, compared with five in the placebo group ($P < 0.001$). No differences among groups were found in visual or hearing impairment. In the conclusion, infants randomized to receive ESA had better cognitive outcomes, compared with placebo recipients, at 18–22 months. Darbe and EPO may prove beneficial in improving long-term cognitive outcomes of preterm infants [166].

The possibility of clinical use of drugs, recombinant EPO to protect the brain, presents the main currently known mechanisms for the implementation of its neuroprotective potential, not connected with the influence on erythropoiesis. Several preclinical and clinical studies have demonstrated that systemic administration of EPO is sufficient to produce behavioral effects. Clinical trials have reported striking improvement in cognitive function in schizophrenia patients and treatment resistant depression. EPO has been shown to improve cognitive function in schizophrenia and treatment resistant depressed patients [162].

However, the potent elevation of red blood cell counts by EPO can cause hematological complications in nonanemic patients. The conducted mass-spectrometry-based peptide mapping of carbamoylated Epo (Cepo) tested its ability to improve cognitive function after social defeat stress. Gene expression analysis in discrete brain regions was performed to obtain mechanistic insight of Cepo action. Cepo reversed stress-induced spatial working memory deficits while affecting long-term (24 h) novel object recognition in these rats. Contextual fear conditioning following defeat was enhanced by Cepo, but attenuated in controls. However, Cepo improved fear extinction in all rats compared to vehicle treatment. Cepo induced differential gene expression of VGF and neuritin in the mPFC and discrete hippocampal subfields, with strongest induction in the dorsal hippocampus. Analysis of gene-brain region-behavior interactions showed that Cepo-induced neurotrophic mechanisms influence cognitive function. Carbamoylated EPO can be developed as a therapeutic neurotrophic agent to treat cognitive dysfunction in neuropsychiatric diseases. Due to its distinct mechanism of action, it is unlikely to cross react with the activity of currently prescribed small molecule drugs and can be used as an add-on biologic drug [167].

The use of EPO in preterm infants both for anemia treatment and correction of immunological and neurological status is considered a prospective direction, but it is complicated by the lack or inconsistency of data on the concentration of endogenous EPO in serum. The concentration of serum EPO in preterm infants with a gestational age of 27–36 weeks and 6 days (Apgar scores 4.32 points) was higher by 1 day after birth and did not differ from a group of full-term infants on 10th day. In preterm infants with gestational age 27–31 weeks and 6 days (Apgar score 3.33), the concentration of serum EPO is higher by 1 day and is lower by 10th day after birth. In preterm infants with gestational age 32–36 weeks and 6 days (Apgar score 5.5), the concentration of serum EPO was lower on 1st day after the birth, and it did not differ from indices in the group of full-term infants on 10th day. The concentration of serum EPO in preterm infants with 27–31 weeks 6 days of gestation increases on the 1st, decreases on 10th day after birth as gestational age decreasing, and the total Apgar score reduces [168].

Pro-cognitive effects of EPO occurred across affective disorders. Neuropsychological screening for cognitive dysfunction may be warranted in future cognition trials.

6. Discussion and conclusions

About one-fifth to one-fourth of children around the world has IDA, in which lack of iron causes problems with hemoglobin—the compound that red blood cells used to transport oxygen through the bloodstream. Many more have low iron without anemia. Children from poor, minority, or immigrant backgrounds are more likely to be ID. ID is associated with alterations in many metabolic processes that may impact brain functioning (e.g., mitochondria electron transport, neurotransmitter synthesis and degradation, protein synthesis, and organogenesis).

Although IDA and ID without anemia may be associated with poor cognitive/behavioral outcomes, this has not been sufficiently studied. In particular, there is lack of dose response studies linking indicators of iron status as continuous risk factors with later cognitive outcomes. The lack of effect in the youngest infants may be because of irreversible effects of ID on the developing brain or the fact that cognitive development and behavior are more difficult to measure in young children [47]. IDA has been consistently linking to altered child affect, energy, and activity, but little knows about how these aberrations affect later development or adjustment in other contexts.

Summarizing the data presented in probably formulates effector mechanisms of influence on the implementation of the ID neurocognitive skills in children and adults:

- hypoxia, tissue hypoxemia
- the enzymatic deficiency in organs of the nervous system and internal environment
- violation of the myelination process, the development of neuropathy
- the development of oxidative stress
- neurodegenerative processes in the central nervous system.

It is extremely difficult to establish a cause-effect relationship between various factors affecting the development of iron deficiency, neurocognitive impairment, and comorbid conditions [2, 11, 20, 36]. For example, it has yet to determine the diagnostic significance of the mutations responsible for the development of severe and/or refractory forms of IDA. Genetic

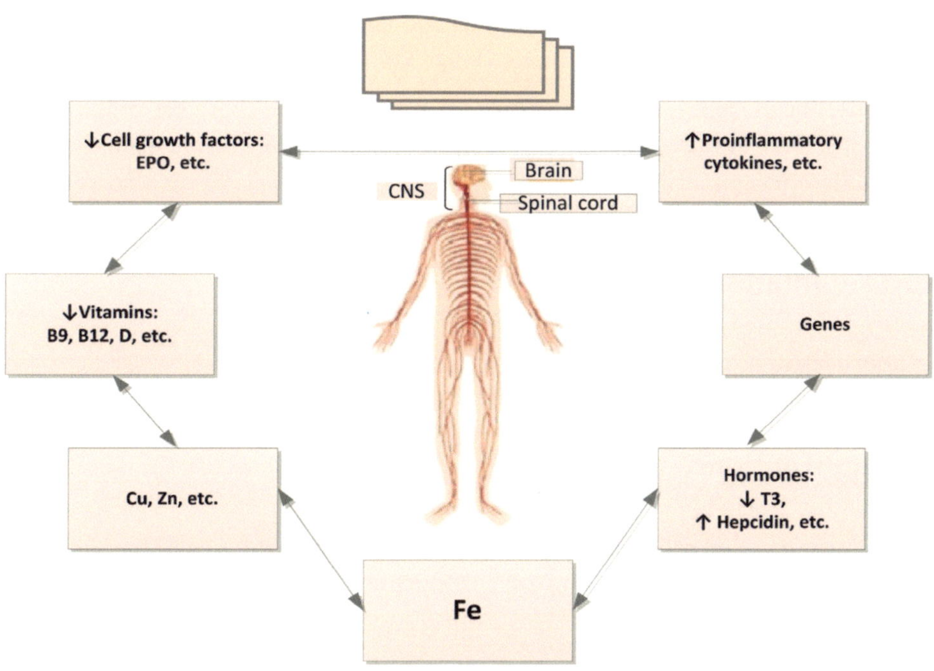

Figure 5. Components of iron homeostasis affecting human neurocognitive development.

causes can involve quantitative or qualitative impairment of globin chain synthesis (thalassemia and sickle cell disease, respectively) [169], or genetically related abnormalities of the erythrocyte, either at the membrane level (pyruvate kinase, glucose-6-phosphate dehydrogenase (G6PD), and stomatocytosis) or concerning enzyme function (hereditary spherocytosis also known as Minkowski-Chauffard syndrome). In addition, a number of rare anemias are related to genetic defects of iron metabolism itself. These defects involve mutations of genes that play a role in systemic or cellular iron metabolism [170]. Despite the relatively low prevalence of iron deficiency in high-income countries using current diagnostic criteria in this healthy cohort, microcytosis was associated with lower cognitive outcomes after 2 years. This research study emphasizes the need to reassess the diagnostic criteria for iron deficiency in young children, while further research is required in studies with adequate nutrition [171].

The metabolic ring of iron homeostasis demonstrates the involvement of a large number of components. However, the establishment of cause-effect relationships is difficult due to differentiate in interpreting the pathogenesis of IDA and cognitive disorders, because of which it is impossible to talk about unidirectional processes in the homeostatic ring of iron (**Figure 5**).

In elderly adults, the cause of cognitive impairment is often vascular lesions of the brain, which can be combined with an imbalance of essential trace elements. Over time, a person begins to show violations of daily behavior due to disruptions in the work of cognitive functions. In children, we need to look mostly for perinatal and post-natal events. So, comprehensive mechanism of the development cognitive dysfunctions in children and elder people needs different protocols for the treatment of ID and IDA.

Difficulties in studying the influence of ID on the level of IQ, individual manifestations of neurocognitive insufficiency, are because they often have a latent character, and in the case of their diagnosis, there are serious problems in deciphering etiology mechanisms and organizing optimal therapy.

Conflicts of interest

The authors declare no conflict of interest.

Author contributions

E. Zhukovskaya retrieved articles, interpreted the results, and drafted and revised the manuscript; A. Karelin contributed in writing the introduction and discussion and interpretation of the findings; and A. Rumyantsev provided critical input to the manuscript and helped with the interpretation of the results.

Author details

Elena Zhukovskaya*, Alexander Karelin and Alexander Rumyantsev

*Address all correspondence to: elena_zhukovskay@mail.ru

Dmitry Rogachev National Research Center of Pediatric Hematology, Oncology and Immunology, Russia

References

[1] Beloshevsky VA. Iron Deficiency in Adults, Children and Pregnant Women. Voronezh: Publ. house named after EA Bolkhovitinova; 2000. 121 p

[2] Sonnweber T, Nairz M, Theurl I, Petzer V, Tymoszuk P, Haschka D, et al. The crucial impact of iron deficiency definition for the course of precapillary pulmonary hypertension. PLoS One. 2018;**13**(8):e0203396. DOI: 10.1371/journal.pone.0203396

[3] Lynch S, Pfeiffer CM, Georgieff MK, Brittenham G, Fairweather-Tait S, Hurrell RF, et al. Biomarkers of nutrition for development (BOND)-iron review. The Journal of Nutrition. 2018;**148**(suppl_1):1001S-1067S. DOI: 10.1093/jn/nxx036

[4] Wieser S, Plessow R, Eichler K, Malek O, Capanzana MV, Agdeppa I, et al. Burden of micronutrient deficiencies by socio-economic strata in children aged 6 months to 5 years in teh Philippines. BMC Public Health. 2013;**13**:1167. DOI: 10.1186/1471-2458-13-1167

[5] Lozoff B, Jimenez E, Wolf AW. Long-term develop mental outcome of infants with iron deficiency. The New England Journal of Medicine. 1991;**325**(10):687-694

[6] Lahat E, Heyman E, Livne A, Goldman M, Berkovitch M, Zachor D, et al. Iron deficiency in children with attention deficit hyperactivity disorder. The Israel Medical Association Journal. 2011;**13**:530-533

[7] Jáuregui-Lobera I. Iron deficiency and cognitive functions. Neuropsychiatric Disease and Treatment. 2014;**10**:2087-2095. DOI: 10.2147/NDT.S72491

[8] Leonard AJ, Chalmers KA, Collins CE, Patterson AJ. A study of the effects of latent iron deficiency on measures of cognition: A pilot randomised controlled trial of iron supplementation in young women. Nutrients. 2014;**6**(6):2419-2435. DOI: 10.3390/nu6062419

[9] Zakharova IN, Dmitrieva YA. Iron deficiency states as a cause of cognitive development disorders in children. Effective Pharmacotherapy. 2012;**33**:42-46

[10] Lozoff B, Jimenez E, Hagen J, Mollen E, Wolf AW. Poorer behavioral and developmental outcome more than 10 years after treatment for iron deficiency in infancy. Pediatrics. 2000;**105**(4):E51

[11] McCann JC, Ames BN. An overview of evidence for a causal relation between iron deficiency during development and deficits in cognitive or behavioral function. The American Journal of Clinical Nutrition. 2007;**85**(4):931-945

[12] Riegler LJ1, Neils-Strunjas J, Boyce S, Wade SL, Scheifele PM. Cognitive intervention results in web-based videophone treatment adherence and improved cognitive scores. Medical Science Monitor. 2013;**19**:269-275. DOI: 10.12659/MSM.883885

[13] Kasatkin VN, Borodina ID, Shurupova MA, Dreneva AA, Ryabova AA, Mironova EV, et al. Correction of executive functions and work of the saccade system in children with bone tumors. Russian Journal of Pediatric Hematology and Oncology. 2017;**4**(3):35-42

[14] Tsuneishi S, Casaer P. Stepwise decrease in VEP latencies and the process of myelination in the human visual pathway. Brain & Development. 1997;**19**:547-551

[15] Tikhomirov AL, Sarsania SI, Nochevkin EV. Some aspects of diagnostics and treatment of iron deficiency states in practical activities at the present stage. Available from: https://medi.ru/info/3470

[16] Iglesias L, Canals J, Arija V. Effects of prenatal iron status on child neurodevelopment and behavior: A systematic review. Critical Reviews in Food Science and Nutrition. 2017;**58**(10):1604-1614. DOI: 10.1080/10408398.2016.1274285

[17] Ru Y, Pressman EK, Guillet R, Katzman PJ, Bacak SJ, O'Brien KO. Predictors of anemia and iron status at birth in neonates born to women carrying multiple fetuses. Pediatric Research. 2018;**84**(2):199-204. DOI: 10.1038/s41390-018-0044-6

[18] McClung J, Murray-KolbIron LE. Nutrition and Premenopausal Women. The Effects of Poor Iron Status on Physical and Neuropsychological Performance Annual Review of Nutrition. 2013;**33**(1):271-288

[19] Hokama T, Gushi Ken M, Nosoko N. Iron deficiency anaemia and child development. Asia-Pacific Journal of Public Health. 2005;**17**(1):19-21

[20] Madhikarmi NL, Murthy KRS. Antioxidant enzymes and oxidative stress in the erythrocytes of iron deficiency anemic patients supplemented with vitamins. Iranian Biomedical Journal. 2014;**18**(2):82-87

[21] Rao R, Georgieff MK. Iron in fetal and neonatal nutrition. Seminars in Fetal & Neonatal Medicine. 2007;**12**:54-63

[22] Chen MH, Su TP, Chen YS, Hsu JW, Huang KL, Chang WH, et al. Association between psychiatric disorders and iron deficiency anemia among children and adolescents: A nationwide population-based study. BMC Psychiatry. 2013;**13**:161

[23] Voloshina NP, Shkorbatov YG, Voloshin-Gaponov IK, Lekomtseva EV, Vazhova EA. Pathogenetic chain of a neurodegenerative process and its clinical manifestations in patients with hepatocerebral dystrophy. Ukrainian Medical Journal. 2014;**6**(104):114-118

[24] Harmony T. Outcome of infants at risk of brain damage after Katona neurohabilitation therapy. International Journal of Neurorehabilitation. 2017;**4**:277. DOI: 10.4172/2376-0281.1000277

[25] Grantham-McGregor S, Ani C. Under nutrition and mental development. Nestle Nutr Workshop Ser Clin Perform Programme. 2001;**5**:1-14; discussion 14-8. Review. The Journal of Nutrition. 2001;**131**(2S-2):649-666

[26] Freedman R, Hunter SK, Hoffman MC. Prenatal primary prevention of mental illness by micronutrient supplements in pregnancy. The American Journal of Psychiatry. 2018;**175**(7):607-619. DOI: 10.1176/appiajp201817070836

[27] Kozlov AV, Gusev EI, Skvortsova VI. Neurology and Neurosurgery. Vol. 1. Moscow: GEOTAR-Media; 2009. p. 624

[28] Ames BN. The metabolic tune-up: Metabolic harmony and disease prevention. The Journal of Nutrition. 2003;**133**:1544S-1548S

[29] Blondel B, Lelong N, Kermarrec M, Goffinet F. Trends in perinatal health in France from 1995 to 2010 results from the French national perinatal surveys. Journal de Gynécologie Obstétrique et Biologie de la Reproduction. 2011;**41**:151-166

[30] Vohr B. Long-term outcomes of moderately preterm, late preterm and early term infants. Clinics in Perinatology. 2013;**40**:739-751

[31] Goodnight W, Newman R. Optimal nutrition for improved twin pregnancy outcome. Obstetrics and Gynecology. 2009;**114**:1121-1134

[32] Allen L. Anemia and iron deficiency: Effects on pregnancy outcome. The American Journal of Clinical Nutrition. 2000;**71**:1280s-1284s

[33] Healthcare in Russia. Stat. Collection of the Russian Statistical Agency—M. 2015. p. 174

[34] Feinstein AR. Pre-therapeutic classification of co-morbidity in chronic disease. Journal of Chronic Diseases. 1970;**23**(7):455-468

[35] Rumyantsev AG, Zakharova IN. Diagnostics and Treatment of Iron Deficiency Anemia in Children and Adolescents. Guideline for Physicians. Moscow: Konti Print Ltd; 2015

[36] Mitchell RM, Simmons Z, Beard JL, Stephens HE, Connor JR. Plasma biomarkers associated with ALS and their relationship to iron homeostasis. Muscle & Nerve. 2010;**42**(1): 95-103

[37] Xu C, Bailly-Maitre B, Reed JC. Endoplasmic reticulum stress: Cell life and death decisions. The Journal of Clinical Investigation. 2005;**115**(10):2656-2664

[38] Kalmijn S, Feskens E, Launer L, Stijnen T, Kromhout D. Glucose intolerance, hyperinsulinaemia and cognitive function in a general population of elderly men. Diabetologia. 1995;**38**(9):1096-1102

[39] Sanna RS, Muthangi S, CS BK, Devi SA. Grape seed proanthocyanidin extract and insulin prevents cognitive decline in type 1 diabetic rat by impacting Bcl-2 and Bax in the prefrontal cortex. Metabolic Brain Disease. 2018:1-15. DOI: 10.1007/s11011-018-0320-5

[40] Saiyasit N, Sripetchwandee J, Chattipakorn N, Chattipakorn SC. Potential roles of neurotensin on cognition in conditions of obese-insulin resistance. Neuropeptides. 2018;**72**: 12-22. DOI: 10.1016/j.npep.2018.09.002

[41] Cheng HL, Bryant C, Cook R, O'Connor H, Rooney K, Steinbeck K. The relationship between obesity and hypoferraemia in adults: A systematic review. Obesity Reviews. 2012;**13**(2):150-161. DOI: 10.1111/j.1467-789X.2011.00938.x

[42] Nead KG, Halterman JS, Kaczorowski JM, Auinger P, Weitzman M. Overweight children and adolescents: A risk group for iron deficiency. Pediatrics. 2004;**114**:104-108. DOI: 10.1542/peds.114.1.104

[43] Nikonorov AA, Tinkov AA, Popova EV, Nemereshina HE, Gatyatulina ER, Skalnaya MG, et al. Iron and obesity: Victim or suspect. Trace Elements in Medicine. 2015;**16**(2):3-9

[44] Grandone A, Marzuillo P, Perrone L, Del Giudice EM. Iron metabolism dysregulation and cognitive dysfunction in pediatric obesity: Is there a connection? Nutrients. 2015;**7**(11): 9163-9170. DOI: 10.3390/nu7115458

[45] Zein S, Rachidi S, Hininger-Favier I. Review. Is oxidative stress induced by iron status associated with gestational diabetes mellitus? Journal of Trace Elements in Medicine and Biology. 2014;**28**(1):65-69

[46] Korovina NA, Zakharova IN, Svintsitskaya VI. Iron Deficiency and Cognitive Disorders in Children. Lechashchiy Vrach. 2006. Available from: http://www.lvrach.ru/2006/05/4533913/

[47] Domello M, Braegger C, Campoy C, Colomb V, Decsi T, Fewtrell M, et al. Iron requirements of infants and toddlers. Journal of Pediatric Gastroenterology and Nutrition. 2014;**58**:119-129

[48] Fonseca C, Araújo M, Moniz P, Marques F, Araújo I, Costa L, et al. Prevalence and prognostic impact of anemia and iron deficiency in patients hospitalized in an internal medicine ward: Teh PRO-IRON study. European Journal of Haematology. 2017;**99**(6):505-513. DOI: 10.1111/ejh.12963

[49] McClung JP, Murray-Kolb LE. Iron nutrition and premenopausal women: The effects of poor iron status on physical and neuropsychological performance. Annual Review of Nutrition. 2013;**33**:271-288. DOI: 10.1146/annurev-nutr-071812-161205

[50] Pulignano G, Del Sindaco D, Di Lenarda A, Tinti MD, Tarantini L, Cioffi G, et al. Chronic renal dysfunction and anaemia are associated with cognitive impairment in older patients with heart failure. Journal of Cardiovascular Medicine. 2014;**15**(6):481-490. DOI: 10.2459/JCM.0000000000000005

[51] Motonishi S, Tanaka K, Ozawa T. Iron deficiency associates with deterioration in several symptoms independently from hemoglobin level among chronic hemodialysis patients. PLoS ONE. 2018;**13**(8):e0201662. https://doi.org/10.1371/journal.pone.0201662

[52] Hidese S, Saito K, Asano S, Kunugi H. Association between iron-deficiency anemia and depression: A web-based Japanese investigation. Psychiatry and Clinical Neurosciences. 2018;**72**(7):513-521. DOI: 10.1111/pcn.12656

[53] Kireeva GN, Bilyalutdinova DI. Investigations of trace elements content in biological substrates in children and adolescents (literature review). Pediatric Bulletin of South Ural. 2015;**2**:58-62

[54] Gordeeva OB, Botvinyeva VV. Modern understanding of iron-deficiency anemia and treatment optimization. Medical Sovet. 2014;**6**:59-65

[55] Oggiano R, Solinas G, Forte G, Bocca B, Farace C, Pisano A, et al. Trace elements in ALS patients and their relationships with clinical severity. Chemosphere. 2018;**197**:457-466. DOI: 10.1016/j.chemosphere.2018.01.076

[56] Pandey S, Pandey SK, Shah V. Role of HAMP genetic variants on pathophysiology of iron deficiency anemia. Indian Journal of Clinical Biochemistry. 2018;**33**(4):479-482. DOI: 10.1007/s12291-017-0707-9

[57] van der Wal HH, van Deursen VM, van der Meer P, Voors AA. Comorbidities in heart failure. Handbook of Experimental Pharmacology. 2017;**243**:35-66. DOI: 10.1007/164_2017_27

[58] Schwartz AJ, Das NK, Ramakrishnan SK, Jain C, Jurkovic M, Wu J, et al. Hepatic hepcidin/intestinal HIF-2α axis maintains iron absorption during iron deficiency and overload. The Journal of Clinical Investigation. 2018;**129**:336-348. DOI: 10.1172/JCI122359

[59] Hallberg L, Rossander L. Effect of different drinks on the absorption of non-heme iron from composite meals. Human Nutrition. Applied Nutrition. 1982;**36**(2):116-123

[60] Bekfani T, Pellicori P, Morris D, Ebner N, Valentova M, Sandek A, et al. Iron deficiency in patients with heart failure wif preserved ejection fraction and its association wif reduced exercise capacity, muscle strength and quality of life. Clinical Research in Cardiology. 2018;**108**(2):203-211. DOI: 10.1007/s00392-018-1344-x

[61] Klimenko LL, Skalny AV, Turna AA, Savostina MS, Mazilina AN, Baskakov IS, et al. Energy metabolism of the brain and the metal-ligand homeostasis in the etiopathogenesis of ischemic stroke. Trace Elements in Medicine. 2015;**16**(2):18-27 [in Russ]

[62] Gusev EI, Kryzhanovsky GN. Dyscirculatory Pathology of the Nervous System. Moscow: Medical Informative Agency; 2009. p. 510

[63] Tolman EC. Cognitive maps in rats and men. Psychological Review. 1948;**55**(4):189-208. DOI: 10.1037/h0061626

[64] Ageeva-Podobed IB, Demyanenko IV, Zhuzhgova IV, Kireeva GN. Rehabilitation of children with cochlear implant. Pediatric Bulletin of South Ural. 2017;**2**:20-24

[65] Inhelder B. Andre Rey. Schweizerische Zeitschrift für Psychologie und ihre Andwendungen. 1965;**24**(3):271-272

[66] Vashura AY, Ryabova AA, Kasatkin VN, Rumyantsev AG. Results of assessment of motor function and nutritional status in children with CNS tumors in remission. Journal of Restorative Medicine & Rehabilitation. 2017;**6**(82):68-74

[67] Iregren A, Gamberale F, Kjellberg A. SPES: A psychological test system to diagnose environmental hazards. Neurotoxicology and Teratology. 1996;**18**:485-491

[68] Resch C, Keulers E, Martens R, van Heugten C, Hurks P. Does strategy instruction on the Rey-Osterrieth complex figure task lead to transferred performance improvement on the

modified taylor complex figure task? A randomized controlled trial in school-aged children. The Clinical Neuropsychologist. 2018;**5**:1-16. DOI: 10.1080/13854046.2018.1448438

[69] Meyers JE, Meyers KR. Rey complex figure test under four different administration procedures. The Clinical Neuropsychologist. 1995;**9**(1):63-67

[70] Konofal E, Lecendreux M, Arnulf I, Mouren MC. Iron deficiency in children with attention-deficit/hyperactivity disorder. Archives of Pediatrics & Adolescent Medicine. 2004;**158**:1113-1115

[71] Loonstra AS, Tarlow AR, Sellers AH. COWAT metanorms across age, education, and gender. Applied Neuropsychology. 2001;**8**(3):161-166. DOI: 10.1207/S15324826AN080

[72] Beery KE, Buktenica NA, Beery NA. Measures the Extent to Which Individuals can Integrate their Visual and Motor Abilities. Available from: https://www.mhs.com/MHS-Assessment?prodname=beeryvmi6

[73] Harvey EM, Leonard-Green TK, Mohan KM, Kulp MT, Davis AL, Miller JM, et al. Interrater and test-retest reliability of the Beery visual-motor integration in school children. Optometry and Vision Science. 2017;**94**(5):598-605. DOI: 10.1097/OPX.0000000000001068

[74] Achenbach TM. Future directions for clinical research, services, and training: Evidence-based assessment across informants, cultures, and dimensional hierarchies. Journal of Clinical Child and Adolescent Psychology. 2017;**46**(1):159-169. DOI: 10.1080/15374416.2016.1220315

[75] Achenbach TM. Advancing assessment of children and adolescents: Commentary on evidence-based assessment of child and adolescent disorders. Journal of Clinical Child and Adolescent Psychology. 2005;**34**(3):541-547

[76] Kasatkin VN, Ryabova AA, Dreneva AA, Rumyantsev AG. Results of the use of battery of Cantab neuropsychological tests for diagnosis of disorders and evaluation of correction of executive functions in children who have transferred complex treatment of postcranial fossa tumors. Bulletin of Restorative Medicine. 2017;**6**(82):3-39

[77] Paul RH, Lawrence J, Williams LM, Richard CC, Cooper N, Gordon E. Preliminary validity of "integneuro^{tm}": A new computerized battery of neurocognitive tests. The International Journal of Neuroscience. 2005;**115**(11):1549-1567. DOI: 10.1080/00207450590957890

[78] Elliot W, Elliot D. Biochemistry and Molecular Biology. Translated from English. Moscow: Institute of Biomedical Chemistry RAMS; 2000. pp. 311-321

[79] Rudisill SS, Martin BR, Mankowski KM, Tessier CR. Iron deficiency reduces synapse formation in the drosophila clock circuit. Biological Trace Element Research. June 2016;**171**(2):237-245. DOI: 10.1007/s12011-018-1442-7

[80] Wilckens KA, Tudorascu DL, Snitz BE, Price JC, Aizenstein HJ, Lopez OL, et al. Sleep moderates the relationship between amyloid beta and memory recall. Neurobiology of Aging. 2018;**71**:142-148. DOI: 10.1016/j.neurobiolaging.2018.07.011

[81] Beard J. Recent evidence from human and animal studies regarding iron status and infant development. The Journal of Nutrition. 2007;**137**:524-530

[82] Coe CL, Lubach GR, Bianco LE, Beard JL. A history of iron deficiency anemia during infancy alters brain monoamine activity later in juvenile monkeys. Developmental Psychobiology. 2009;**51**:301-309

[83] Levi S, Taveggia C. Iron homeostasis in peripheral nervous system, still a black box? Antioxidants & Redox Signaling. 2014;**21**(4):634-648. DOI: 10.1089/ars.2013.5813

[84] Skalny AV, Rudakov IA. Bioelements in Medicine. Moscow: House Onyx; 2004. 272 p

[85] Natural Ways to Increase Myelin Sheath + Function & Facts. Neuroscience. 2018. Available from: https://www.selfhacked.com/blog/myelin/

[86] Nave KA, Trapp BD. Axonglial signaling and the glial support of axon function. Annual Review of Neuroscience. 2008;**31**:535-556

[87] Yager JY, Hartfield DS. Neurologic manifestations of iron deficiency in childhood. Pediatric Neurology. 2002;**27**:85-92

[88] Calarge C, Farmer C, DiSilvestro R, Arnold LE. Serum ferritin and amphetamine response in youth with attention-deficit/hyperactivity disorder. Journal of Child and Adolescent Psychopharmacology. 2010;**20**:495-502

[89] Berthold CH, Fraher K, King RHM, Rydmark MJP. Microscopic anatomy of the peripheral nervous system. In: Peripheral Neuropathy, edited by Dyck PJ, editor; and Thomas PK. Philadelphia, PA: Saunders, 2005. pp. 35-80

[90] Zalc B, Colman DR. Origins of vertebrate success. Science. 2000;**288**:271-272

[91] Earley CJ, Connor J, Garcia-Borreguero D, Jenner P, Winkelman J, Zee PC, et al. Altered brain iron homeostasis and dopaminergic function in restless legs syndrome (Willis-Ekbom disease). Sleep Medicine. 2014;**15**(11):1288-1301

[92] Allen RP. Restless leg syndrome/Willis-Ekbom disease pathophysiology. Sleep Medicine Clinics. 2015;**10**(3):207-214

[93] Wijemanne S, Jankovic J. Restless legs syndrome: Clinical presentation diagnosis and treatment. Sleep Medicine. 2015;**16**(6):678-690

[94] Li X, Allen RP, Earley CJ, Liu H, Cruz TE, Edden RAE, et al. Brain iron deficiency in idiopathic restless legs syndrome measured by quantitative magnetic susceptibility at 7 tesla. Sleep Medicine. 2016;**22**:75-82

[95] Peirano PD, Calgarín CA, Garrido MI, Pediatr LB. Iron deficiency anemia in infancy is associated with altered temporal organization of sleep states in childhood. Pediatric Research. 2007;**62**(6):715-719

[96] Fallone G, Owens JA, Deane J. Sleepiness in children and adolescents: Clinical implications. Sleep Medicine Reviews. 2002;**6**:287-306

[97] Algarin C, Peirano P, Garrido M, Pizarro FA, Lozoff B. Iron Deficiency Anemia (IDA) in infancy alters the temporal organization of sleep states in childhood. April 2001;**24**:A13-A13

[98] Otero G, Fernandez T, Bernardo F, Mendieta GG. Among iron-deficient anemic infants. Nutritional Neuroscience. 2019;**22**(5):363-372. DOI: 10.1080/1028415X.2017.1391529

[99] Tran PV, Fretham SJ, Carlson ES, Georgieff MK. Long-term reduction of hippocampal brain-derived neurotrophic factor activity after fetal-neonatal iron deficiency in adult rats. Pediatric Research. 2009;**65**:493-498

[100] Blegen MB, Kennedy BC, Thibert KA, Gewirtz JC, Tran PV, Georgieff MK. Multi-generational effects of fetal-neonatal iron deficiency on hippocampal BDNF signaling. Physiological Reports. 2013;**1**(5):e00096

[101] Kaller MS, Lazari A, Blanco-Duque C, Sampaio-Baptista C, Johansen-Berg H. Myelin plasticity and behaviour-connecting the dots. Current Opinion in Neurobiology. 2017;**47**:86-92. DOI: 10.1016/j.conb.2017.09.014

[102] Lozoff B, Beard J, Connor J, Barbara F, Georgieff M, Schallert T. Long-lasting neural and behavioral effects of iron deficiency in infancy. Nutrition Reviews. 2006;**64**:S34-S91

[103] Mochizuki Y, Go T, Ohkubo H, Tatara T, Motomura T. Developmental changes of brain-stem auditory evoked potentials (BAEPs) in normal human subjects from infants to young adults. Brain & Development. 1982;**4**:127-136

[104] Algarin C, Peirano P, Garrido M, Pizarro F, Lozoff B. Iron deficiency anemia in infancy: Long-lasting effects on auditory and visual systems functioning. Pediatric Research. 2003;**53**:217-223

[105] Belaidi AA, Bush AI. Iron neurochemistry in Alzheimer's disease and Parkinson's disease: Targets for therapeutics. Journal of Neurochemistry. 2016;**139**(Suppl 1):179-197. DOI: 10.1111/jnc.13425

[106] Youdim MB. Brain iron deficiency and excess: Cognitive impairment and neurodegeneration with involvement of striatum and hippocampus. Neurotoxicity Research. 2008;**14**:45-56

[107] Carlson ES, Tkac I, Magid R, O'Connor MB, Andrews NC, Schallert T, et al. Iron is essential for neuron development and memory function in mouse hippocampus. The Journal of Nutrition. 2009;**139**:672-679

[108] Barks A, Fretham SJB, Georgieff MK, Tran PV. Life neuronal-specific iron deficiency alters teh adult mouse hippocampal transcriptome. The Journal of Nutrition. 2018;**148**(10): 1521-1528. DOI: 10.1093/jn/nxy125

[109] Erikson KM, Jones BC, Beard JL. Iron deficiency alters dopamine transporter functioning in rat striatum. The Journal of Nutrition. 2000;**130**:2831-2837

[110] Rao R, Tkac I, Townsend EL, Gruetter R, Georgieff MK. Perinatal iron deficiency alters the neurochemical profile of the developing rat hippocampus. The Journal of Nutrition. 2003;**133**:3215-3221

[111] Haschka D, Volani C, Stefani A, Tymoszuk P, Mitterling T, Holzknecht E, et al. Idiopathic restless legs syndrome association of mitochondrial iron deficiency and dysfunction with idiopathic restless legssyndrome. Movement Disorders. 2018. DOI: 10.1002/mds. 27482

[112] Islam K, Seth S, Saha S, Roy A, Das R, Datta AK. A study on association of iron deficiency with attention deficit hyperactivity disorder in a tertiary care center. Indian Journal of Psychiatry. 2018;**60**(1):131-134. DOI: 10.4103/psychiatry.IndianJPsychiatry_197_17

[113] Juneja M, Jain R, Singh V, Mallika V. Iron deficiency in Indian children with attention deficit hyperactivity disorder. Indian Pediatrics. 2010;**47**:955-958

[114] Sever Y, Ashkenazi A, Tyano S, Weizman A. Iron treatment in children with attention deficit hyperactivity disorder. A preliminary report. Neuropsychobiology. 1997;**35**: 178-180

[115] Kwon HJ, Lim MH, Ha M, Kim EJ, Yoo SJ, Kim JW, et al. Transferrin in Korean children with attention deficit hyperactivity disorder. Psychiatry Investigation. 2011;**8**:366-371

[116] Maguire JL, deVeber G, Parkin PS. Association between iron-deficiency anemia and stroke in young children. Pediatrics. 2007;**120**(5):1053-1057

[117] Son SJ, Lee KS, Na DL, Seo SW, Kim CH, Kim JH, et al. The effect of anemia and white matter hyperintensities (WMH) on cognitive impairment in patients with amnestic mild cognitive impairment (MCI). Archives of Gerontology and Geriatrics. 2012;**55**(2):251-256. DOI: 10.1016/j.archger.2011.10. 015

[118] Beard J. One person's vie of iron deficiency, development, and cognitive function. The American Journal of Clinical Nutrition. 1995;**62**:709-710

[119] Roncagliolo M, Garrido M, Walter T, Peirano P, Lozoff B. Evidence of altered central nervous system development in infants with iron deficiency anemia at 6 months: Delayed maturation of auditory brainstem responses. The American Journal of Clinical Nutrition. 1998;**68**(3):683-690

[120] Kretchmer N, Beard JL, Carlson S. The role of nutrition in the development of normal cognition. The American Journal of Clinical Nutrition. 1996;**63**:997S-1001S

[121] Del Aguila CM, Nunez O. Controlled trial of maltofer (iron(III)-hydroxide polymaltose complex) vs. ferinsol (ferrous sulphate) in the treatment of iron deficiency anemia in children aged from 6 months to 2 years. Revista del Awgla. 2007;**3**:28-39

[122] Rao R, Tkac I, Townsend EL, Ennis K, Gruetter R, Georgieff MK. Perinatal iron deficiency predisposes the developing rat hippocampus to greater injury from mild to moderate hypoxia-ischemia. Journal of Cerebral Blood Flow and Metabolism. 2007;**27**:872

[123] Ward KL, Tkac I, Jing Y, Felt B, Beard J, Connor J, et al. Gestational and lactational iron deficiency alters the developing striatal metabolome and associated behaviors in young rats. The Journal of Nutrition. 2007;**137**:1043-1049

[124] Fretham SJB, Carlson ES, Georgieff MK. The role of iron in learning and memory. Advances in Nutrition. 2011;**2**(2):112-121. DOI: 10.3945/an.110.000190

[125] Carter RC, Jacobson JL, Burden MJ, Armony-Sivan R, Dodge NC, Angelilli ML, et al. Iron deficiency anemia and cognitive function in infancy. Iron deficiency anemia and cognitive function in infancy. Pediatrics. 2010;**126**(2):e427-e434. DOI: 10.1542/peds.2009-2097

[126] Lozoff B, Clark KM, Jing Y, Armony-Sivan R, Angelilli ML, Jacobson SW. Dose-response relationships between iron deficiency with or without anemia and infant social-emotional behavior. The Journal of Pediatrics. 2008;**152**(5):696-702

[127] Thorisdottir AV, Gunnarsdottir I, Palsson GI, Gretarsson SJ, Thorsdottir I. Iron status and developmental scores in 6-year-olds highlights ongoing need to tackle iron deficiency in infants. Acta Paediatrica. 2013;**102**(9):914-919. DOI: 10.1111/apa.12316

[128] Lozoff B. Early iron deficiency has brain and behavior effects consistent with dopaminergic dysfunction. The Journal of Nutrition. 2011;**141**(4):740S-746S

[129] Iron deficiency, lower cognitive scores Iron deficiency, lower cognitive scores. Internet: https://www.upi.com/Iron-deficiency-lower-cognitive-scores/88781163013940/

[130] Leonard AJ, Chalmers KA, Collins CE, Patterson AJ. A study of the effects of latent iron deficiency on measures of cognition: A pilot randomized controlled trial of iron supplementation in young women. Nutrients. 2014;**6**(6):2419-2435. DOI: 10.3390/nu6062419

[131] Suranova NV. Failure of attention in children and its relation to sideropenia. Series: Medical and Biological Sciences. Vestnik of Northern (Arctic) Federal University. 2014;**1**: 105-107 (in Russ)

[132] Rakesh PS, Rajeswaran T, Rakesh R, Gigil M, Sheeja AL, Subhagan S. Anemia among schoolchildren from southern Kerala folic acid, India. A cross-sectional study. National Medical Journal of India. 2015;**28**(5):225-227

[133] East P, Lozoff B, Blanco E, Delker E, Delva J, Encina P, et al. Iron deficiency, child affect, and maternal unresponsiveness: Testing the long-term effects of functional isolation [Internet]. Developmental Psychology. 2017. DOI: 10.1037/dev0000385

[134] Kebede A, Gerensea H, Amare F, Tesfay Y, Teklay G. The magnitude of anemia and associated factors among pregnant women attending public institutions of Shire Town, Shire, Tigray, Northern Ethiopia, 2018. BMC Research Notes. 2018;**11**(1):595. DOI: 10.1186/s13104-018-3706-x

[135] Grantham-McGregor SM, Ani CC. The role of micronutrients in psychomotor and cognitive development. British Medical Bulletin. 1999;**55**:511-527

[136] Gromova OA, Torshin IY, Khadzhidis AK. Analysis of molecular mechanisms of iron (II), copper, manganese impact in pathogenesis of iron deficiency anemia. Clinical Pharmacology and Pharmacoekonomy. 2010;**1**:1-9

[137] Skalny AV. Chemical Elements in Human Physiology and Ecology. Moscow: House MIR; 2004. 216 p

[138] Singh M. Role of micronutrients for physical growth and mental development. Indian Journal of Pediatrics. 2004;**71**(1):59-62

[139] Zeglam A, Abugrara A, Kabuka M. Autosomal-recessive iron deficiency anemia, dystonia and hypermanganesemia caused by new variant mutation of the manganese transporter gene SLC39A14. Acta Neurologica Belgica. 19 September 2018:1-6. DOI: 10.1007/s13760-018-1024-7

[140] Bremner I, Dalgarno AC. Iron metabolism in the veal calf. The British Journal of Nutrition. 1973;**30**:61-76

[141] Wasantwisut E. Nutrition and development: Other micronutrients' effect on growth and cognition. The Southeast Asian Journal of Tropical Medicine and Public Health. 1997;**28**(Suppl 2):78-82

[142] Bird LJ, Coleman ML, Newman DK. Iron and copper act synergistically to delay anaerobic growth of bacteria. Applied and Environmental Microbiology. 2013;**79**(12):3619-3627. DOI: 10.1128/AEM.03944-12

[143] Liu J, Hanlon A, Ma C, Zhao SR, Cao S, Compher C. Low blood zinc, iron, and other sociodemographic factors associated with behavior problems in preschoolers. Nutrients. 2014;**6**(2):530-545

[144] Wang X, Flores SRL, Ha J-H, Doguer C, Woloshun RR, Xiang P, et al. Intestinal DMT1 is essential for optimal assimilation of dietary copper in male and female mice with iron-deficiency anemia. The Journal of Nutrition. 2018;**148**(8):1244-1252. DOI: 10.1093/jn/nxy111

[145] Sayre LM, Perry G, Atwood CS, Smith MA. The role of metals in neurodegenerative diseases. Cellular and Molecular Biology. 2000;**46**(4):731-741

[146] Hallberg L, Rossander L, Persson H, Svahn E. Deleterious effects of prolonged warming of meals on ascorbic acid content and iron absorption. The American Journal of Clinical Nutrition. 1982;**36**(5):846-850. DOI: 10.1093/ajcn/36.5.846

[147] Pollitt E. The developmental and probabilistic nature of the functional consequences of iron-deficiency anemia in children. The Journal of Nutrition. 2001;**131**:669S-675S

[148] Sarsaniya SI, Tihomirov AL, Nochevkin EV, Tuskaev KS. Nuances of diagnosis and treatment of asiderotic anemia. Difficult patient. 2012;**2-3**:23-34

[149] Skalny AV, Grabeklis AR, Tinkov AA, Nikonorov AA, Zhukovskaya EV, Kireeva GN, et al. Whole blood and hair trace elements and minerals in children living in metal-polluted area near copper smelters in Karabash Chelyabinsk region Russia. Environmental Science and Pollution Research. 2017;**24**(3):2014-2020

[150] Lee JA, Hwang JS, Hwang IT, Kim DH, Seo JH, Lim JS. Low vitamin D levels are associated with both iron deficiency and anemia in children and adolescents. Pediatric Hematology and Oncology. 2015;**32**(2):99-108. DOI: 10.3109/08880018.2014.983623

[151] Chowdhury R, Taneja S, Bhandari N, Strand TA, Bhan MK. Vitamin D deficiency and mild to moderate anemia in young North Indian children: A secondary data analysis. Nutrition. 2018;**57**:63-68. DOI: 10.1016/j.nut. 2018.05.034

[152] Enderami A, Zarghami M, Darvishi-Khezri H. The effects and potential mechanisms of folic acid on cognitive function: A comprehensive review. Neurological Sciences. 2018;**39**(10):1667-1675. DOI: 10.1007/s10072-018-3473-4

[153] Mooijaart SP, Gussekloo J, Frölich M, Jolles J, Stott DJ, Westendorp RCJ, et al. Homocysteine, vitamin B-12, and folic acid and the risk of cognitive decline in old age: the Leiden 85-Plus Study. The American Journal of Clinical Nutrition. 2005;**82**(4):866-871. DOI: 10.1093/ajcn/82.4.866

[154] Brines M, Cerami A. Emerging biological roles for erythropoietin in the nervous system. Nature Reviews. Neuroscience. 2005;**6**:484-494. DOI: 10.1038/nrn1687

[155] Azmandian J, Abbasi MR, Pourfarziani V, Nasiri AA, Ossareh S, Ezzatzadegan Jahromi S, et al. Comparing therapeutic efficacy and safety of epoetin beta and epoetin alfa in teh treatment of anemia in end-stage renal disease hemodialysis patients. American Journal of Nephrology. 2018;**48**(4):251-259. DOI: 10.1159/000493097

[156] Tubiana M. Mechanisms of increasing the proliferation of hematopoietic cells. Growth factors and inhibitors. Historical perspectives. Bulletin de l'Académie Nationale de Médecine. 1994;**178**(5):739-748

[157] Ma C, Cheng F, Wang X, et al. Erythropoietin pathway: A potential target for the treatment of depression. International Journal of Molecular Sciences. 2016;**17**(5):E677

[158] Osborn M, Rustom N, Clarke M, Litteljohn D, Rudyk C, Anisman H, et al. Antidepressant-like effects of erythropoietin: A focus on behavioral and hippocampal processes. PLoS One. 2013;**8**(9):e72813. DOI: 10.1371/journal.pone.007281

[159] Sathyanesan M, Watt MJ, Haiar JH, Scholl JL, Davies DR, Paulsen RT, et al. Carbamoylated erythropoietin modulates cognitive outcomes of social defeat and differentially regulates gene expression in the dorsal and ventral hippocampus. Translational Psychiatry. 2018;**8**:113. DOI: 10.1038/s41398-018-0168-9

[160] Bunn HF. Erythropoietin. Cold Spring Harbor Perspectives in Medicine. 2013;**3**(3): a011619. DOI: 10.1101/cshperspect.a011619

[161] Ott CV, Vinberg M, Kessing LV, Miskowiak KW. The effect of erythropoietin on cognition in affective disorders—associations with baseline deficits and change in subjective cognitive complaints. European Neuropsychopharmacology. 2016;**26**(8):1264-1273. DOI: 10.1016/j.euroneuro.2016.05.009

[162] Bekker RA, Bykov YV. On the Role of Neuroendocrine Abnormalities in the Pathogenesis of Cognitive Dysfunction in Major Depressive Disorder (A Literature Review with Authors' Comments). Available from: http://con-med.ru/partner_article/all/o-roli-neyroendokrinnykh-narusheniy-vpatogeneze-kognitivnoy-disfunktsii-pri-depressivnykhb-sostoyani

[163] Girgenti MJ, Hunsberger J, Duman CH, Sathyanesan M, Terwilliger R, Newton SS. Erythropoietin induction by electroconvulsive seizure, gene regulation, and antidepressant-like behavioral effects. Biological Psychiatry. 2009;**66**:267-274. DOI: 10.1016/j.biopsych. 2008. 12.005

[164] Kellner CH, Adams DA, Benferhat A. Further improving the cognitive effect profile of electroconvulsive therapy (ECT): The case for studying carbamylated erythropoietin. Medical Hypotheses. 2015;**84**(3):258-261

[165] Patel S, Ohls RK. Darbepoetin administration in term and preterm neonates. Clinics in Perinatology. 2015;**42**(3):557-566. DOI: 10.1016/j.clp.2015.04.016

[166] Ohls RK, Kamath-Rayne BD, Christensen RD, Wiedmeier SE, Rosenberg A, Fuller J, et al. Cognitive outcomes of preterm infants randomized to darbepoetin, erythropoietin, or placebo. Pediatrics. 2014;**133**(6):1023-1030. DOI: 10.1542/peds.2013-4307

[167] Osikov MV, Almukhametova ON, Klimova EV, Fetisov AA. Concentration of blood erythropoietin in preterm infants. Current Problem of Science and Education. 2015;**3**:234

[168] Li S, Gao X, Wei Y, Zhu G, Yang C. The relationship between iron deficiency and thyroid function in Chinese women during early pregnancy. Journal of Nutritional Science and Vitaminology (Tokyo). 2016;**62**(6):397-401. DOI: 10.3177/jnsv. 62. 397

[169] Sanger M, Jordan L, Pruthi S, Day M, Covert B, Merriweather B, et al. Cognitive deficits are associated with unemployment in adults with sickle cell anemia. Journal of Clinical and Experimental Neuropsychology. 2016;**38**(6):661-671. DOI: 10.1080/13803395.2016.1149153

[170] Brissot P, Bernard D, Brissot E, Loreal O, M-Berengere T. Rare anemias due to genetic iron metabolism defects. Mutation Research, Reviews in Mutation Research. 2018;**777**: 52-63. DOI: 10.1016/j.mrrev.2018.06.003

[171] McCarthy E, Kiely M, Hannon G, Ahearne C, Kenny L, Hourihane J, et al. Microcytosis is associated with low cognitive outcomes in healthy 2-year-olds in a high-resource setting. The British Journal of Nutrition. 2017;**118**(5):360-367. DOI: 10.1017/S0007114517001945